# YOUR HIP
# REPLACEMENT

# YOUR HIP REPLACEMENT

## A Patient's Guide To:

Understanding Hip Arthritis
Preparing for Surgery
Maximizing Your Outcome

## Ryan C. Koonce, MD

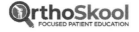

OrthoSkool
FOCUSED PATIENT EDUCATION

Published in the United States of America

Cover design by David Litwin / Pure Fusion Media
Cover image © [Sebastian Kaulitzki] / Adobe Stock

# Why You Should Read This Book

The modern hip replacement was developed in the 1960s. Since that time, it has revolutionized the treatment of crippling arthritis and has improved the lives of millions of patients.

Over the last six decades, we have seen significant advancements in the quality of hip surgery, but the results are far from perfect. Patients can influence the success of their surgery by arming themselves with knowledge. Determining whether hip replacement is right for you, finding the right surgeon, preparing for surgery, and following recovery rules all affect your chances of a quality outcome.

As a surgeon whose been specializing in treating hip arthritis for nearly a decade, I have been searching for a trusted, unbiased, and up-to-date source of patient education materials to help guide my patients through the journey of hip replacement. Unsatisfied with what I found; I created my own book. This book contains proven education and messaging backed by thousands of successful outcomes. It will help you, your family member, or your friend through this complex yet navigable process.

Also by Ryan C. Koonce, MD:

*YOUR KNEE REPLACEMENT*
*A Patient Guide To:*
*Understanding Knee Arthritis*
*Preparing for Surgery*
*Maximizing Your Outcome*

*NON-SURGICAL TREATMENT OPTIONS*
*FOR KNEE OSTEOARTHRITIS*

*NON-SURGICAL TREATMENT OPTIONS*
*FOR HIP OSTEOARTHRITIS*

_____

For online joint replacement education, check out:
www.OrthoSkool.com

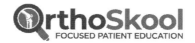

# Contents

## Appendix

This book is dedicated to my wonderful family.
To my parents, Hal and Pat. To Nathan, Anna, Nick, Carolyn,
and my extended Koonce, Krohn, and Shudra families.

To you all, I echo the words of my beloved mother:
*"Synonyms for love are affection, attachment, devotion, and fondness.
I feel all of these for you, but love is still the best word."*

*Patricia Ann Koonce Cole*
*1947 - 1997*

# Acknowledgments

I sincerely appreciate the surgeons who patiently trained me in the science and art of orthopedic surgery. To the surgeons at the *University of Colorado*, who reinforced the critical concept of putting patients first, and later welcomed me home as a colleague. To the surgeons at *San Diego Sports Medicine and Arthroscopy Fellowship*, who showed me the joy in caring for active patients. To the surgeons at the renowned *Anderson Orthopaedic Clinic*, who humbled me with their knowledge, inspired me with their intellect, and shared their exceptional surgical techniques. Thank you doesn't cover it.

My four patient education books would not have materialized without the invaluable editorial skills of Susan Strecker and the typesetting expertise of Sue Balcer. Thank you for your professionalism, contributions, and patience with this humble author.

Lastly, thank you to the patients, past, present and future, who put their trust in me as their surgeon. It is an honor and a privilege to be part of your joint replacement journey.

Chapter One

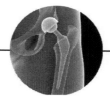

# Introduction

"Steve" is a retired executive turned rancher. After a long and prosperous career sitting at a desk, enduring countless meetings, and working late under fluorescent lights, he wanted his retirement to be active and outdoors. He purchased a ranch in the mountains of Colorado where he worked in the sun harvesting hay and tending to livestock. He loved walking his property lines and mending barbed wire fence. Compared to his prior office job, Steve achieved what many hope to accomplish in retirement – he was active, healthy, and content.

A couple years into his new-found life, Steve noticed pain around his right hip. At first, he controlled it with over-the-counter pain relievers. With time, he was unable to make it through a full workday because his hip ached with every step. He saw his primary care doctor who ordered a cortisone injection into the hip joint. This helped him for six months, but the pain returned worse than ever.

Steve came to see me when his ability to maintain his ranch was severely compromised. His x-rays showed that all the cartilage was worn away in his hip joint. Surgery was something that he preferred to avoid, but he was willing to take on any treatment that would return his ability to work on the ranch. After discussing his options, we decided to proceed with hip replacement surgery.

Steve had lots of questions about the surgery process and wanted a definitive plan to follow. Like most patients, he wanted to do everything in his power to achieve a successful outcome. I believe that Steve's interest and investment in his own care played a large role in what was a fantastic outcome that allowed him to resume all ranching duties.

This book was written to empower patients and their loved ones to navigate the process of hip replacement surgery. You will be armed with information that will allow you to speak the language of hip arthritis, understand your treatment options, and, should you choose to move forward with hip replacement surgery, it will help you maximize your outcome.

## Finding the Right Information

Mild hip pain may take the fun out of your normal leisure activities. Severe pain can make basic tasks such as standing, walking, and sleeping challenging. It's surprising how your overall quality of life might be connected to a single painful joint.

Physicians often do a poor job of providing trustworthy educational resources to our patients. It is not economically feasible for medical providers to sit down and educate patients one-on-one about the intricate details of hip replacement surgery. There is so much to cover on the topic that patients will need more than just a doctor's visit to properly prepare.

Have you ever found yourself asking "Dr. Google", as we refer to Internet medical advice, for information about a symptom you are experiencing? You are not alone. Millions of Americans turn to the Internet for help before making critical decisions about their health or the health of someone they love.

Unfortunately, searching for random information on the Internet can pose a risk to your health as many available resources are misleading. "Dr. Google" might be more of a foe than a friend. In addition to the Internet, you will find a variety of inaccurate media, outdated books, and seemingly knowledgeable family, friends, and professionals who are ready to offer their advice. You truly have to be careful about people or resources posing as subject-matter experts.

The ultimate goal of this book is to help you make the best decisions. The advice you will read here is the culmination of nearly two decades of education, training, experience, and keen observation of patients being treated for hip pain. I have watched thousands of patients undergo non-operative and operative treatments for hip conditions, and I have witnessed their outcomes.

1. Those who have hip pain and are wondering if hip replacement might be a solution for them.

2. Those who are in the process of planning a hip replacement procedure and want the best possible outcome.

## Hip Replacement is Your Unique Journey

An instant fix or a quick drive-through meal – these are the norms in our culture. We want to press a button and let the machine give us an immediate answer. These days, we don't even have to press a button. We can just yell, "Hey, Alexa" or "Okay, Google" and these virtual assistants will get the job done.

We also want an instant fix to our health issues. We want a pill, injection, or procedure that resolves any health condition immediately. Unfortunately, there are only a few medical conditions where a quick fix is the answer, and hip arthritis is not one of them.

When this book talks about "hip replacement", it is not referring to a procedure, but rather, a process or a journey. Your journey starts the day you seek medical treatment for hip arthritis and ends when you are satisfied with the final result of your treatment and you resume the activities you enjoy. You will learn that this process can take months, maybe even a year. And if you choose to embark on this journey, you will experience it differently than everyone else.

Imagine you have a friend who recalls a trip of a lifetime to Europe last year. He told you all about his trip, recommended which hotels and sites to visit or avoid, and how to find the best bangers and mash, croissants, and wiener schnitzel. You decide to pack up your suitcase and repeat your friend's magical trip. I can assure you, that even if your itinerary is identical on paper, your *experience* will be different. Hip replacement is like this. The human experience is a combination of personal history, our upbringing, DNA, emotions, sensations, expectations, and uncontrollable outside variables. The purpose of this book is to help optimize the parts you can control and understand the parts that you cannot.

## How to Use This Book

This book is broken into sections based on patient needs. You only need to read as far as your personal journey takes you.

Chapters 1 –4          For patients looking to understand knee ar-
                       thritis and basics of non-operative treatment
                       options.

Chapters 5 – 6         For patients who understand the information in
                       Chapters 1–3 but are on the fence about moving
                       forward with knee replacement surgery. These
                       chapters explain the surgery itself, the risks,
                       and the benefits.

Chapters 7 – 12        For those who understand the information in
                       Chapters 1-5 and have decided that knee re-
                       placement is necessary.

This book contains some references. I've tried to reference only topics where the author or publisher deserves credit. Any topic for which I have not provided a reference should be considered my understanding of the subject based on my training, research, and successful experiences with patients.

Learning about a medical condition and associated treatments is akin to learning a new language. For this reason, many medical terms are placed in *italics* and have definitions in the Glossary.

## What This Book is Not

This book provides honest and accurate information. Every surgeon has different training backgrounds, sources of information, and patient care experiences. I base the information on what most joint replacement surgeons would agree with. This book represents information that I recommend other surgeons follow in their practice, but your own surgeon may have different preferences.

This book will not address the complex issue of pain in existing hip replacements or provide in-depth coverage of complications associated with hip replacements. If you have already had a hip replacement and are looking for solutions for ongoing pain or other problems, please consult a local joint replacement surgeon
oint replacement surgeon.

## Conflicts of Interest

The author and publisher have no conflicts of interest or paid relationships with medical device companies, drug companies, or any other financial incentives that would cause us to recommend specific surgical and non-surgical treatment options. Any potential conflicts of interest that might arise after the publication date of this book will be disclosed on www.orthoskool.com.

## Chapter 1 Review

- There is a lot of information out there. Obtaining the right information is critical to understanding hip pain, arthritis, and treatment options.

- Hip replacement is not a single procedure, it's a journey.

- Everyone experiences hip pain and hip replacement surgery differently.

- Preparation and education will enhance your experience and your outcome, whether you have a hip replacement or choose a non-operative treatment.

Chapter Two

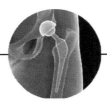

# The Basics of Hip Arthritis
## *The Burdensome Hip*

If you have *chronic* hip pain, you probably remember a time when you were pain-free. As children and teenagers, most of us were very active and were not limited by joint pain. Some describe the feeling of their youth as "invincible". We could run, jump, skip, pivot, cut, and dance for hours without pain. Our hips were no different than our earlobe in that that it was a body part and not a pain generator. If you have hip arthritis, it's possible that you are aware of your hip joint every day, maybe with every step.

In this chapter, we define normal anatomy, the condition of arthritis, and describe how the invincible hip became the burdensome hip. With these building blocks in place, we will have the background to discuss treatment options in upcoming chapters.

## Hip Anatomy—The Invincible Hip Before Arthritis

We are going to stick to the basics, but there is some anatomy you must understand about the normal hip before we move on to what went wrong. The hip is what is referred to as a *ball and socket* joint. The structure of the joint allows for a wide range of motion.

The hip joint is made up of 2 bones (Figure 2-1):

1. *Femur*: Your thigh bone. The longest bone in the body, extending from your hip joint to your knee joint. The top part of the femur forms the ball part of the ball and socket joint. The round ball is called the *femoral head,* and the segment that connects the head to the rest of the femur is called the *femoral neck.*

2.  *Bony pelvis*: Your bony pelvis makes up the socket side of the hip joint. The socket itself is called the *acetabulum*. The acetabulum is a hemispherical cavity that is approximately the same size and shape as the femoral head. The femoral head and acetabulum mate to form the hip joint.

There are several soft tissue structures surrounding the hip joint that include *muscles, tendons, and ligaments*. These help to hold the femoral head in the socket. Most of these structures are not critical for understanding the development and treatment of hip arthritis. Two soft tissues that play a role in arthritis are *articular cartilage* (which is the surface cartilage that protects the ball and the socket), and the *labrum*. Think of the articular cartilage as a smooth and slick surface that allows the ball to glide around easily within the socket. The labrum is tough, fibrous cartilage that follows the rim of the socket and serves to cushion and seal the joint.

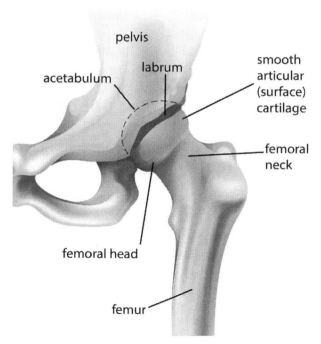

**Figure 2-1**: Bones and cartilage that make up the hip joint. This is a ball and socket joint made up of the femoral head (ball) and acetabulum (socket).

# Hip Arthritis—The Burdensome Hip

The Greek word *arthron* means "joint". The condition of inflammation is described in medicine with the suffix *-itis*. Combine these to form the word *arthr-itis* in English which simply means "inflamed joint", just like *col-itis* is an inflamed colon, and *bronch-itis* is inflammation in the bronchi of your lungs. An additional descriptor that I would add for the condition of hip arthritis is "cartilage wear". The few millimeters of cartilage that cover the ends of the bone are often worn away leaving exposed bone underneath. This cartilage wear causes inflammation and pain. Most patients with arthritis also tear the labrum inside the joint. Figure 2-2 shows an arthritic hip joint.

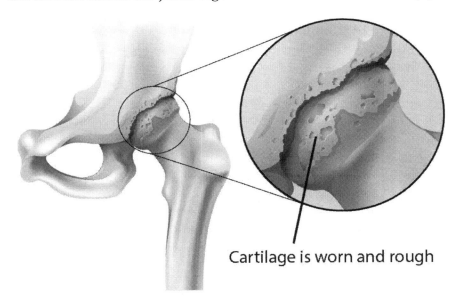

## Cartilage is worn and rough

**Figure 2-2**: The arthritic hip is shown. Note that the normally smooth cartilage surfaces are worn and rough.

The definitive test to diagnose hip arthritis is the x-ray (Figure 2-3). There are several criteria used to make the diagnosis, but the three most common are:

1.  *Cartilage space narrowing*: Bone shows up on an x-ray. Cartilage is transparent on x-ray. Narrowing of the space where cartilage used to be is the x-ray sign of cartilage wear.

2.  *Osteophytes*: These are outcroppings of bone and/or cartilage on the edge of the hip joint, commonly known as "bone spurs". These spurs **do not cause arthritis**. The cartilage wear causes them to form over time.

3.  *Bone cysts:* These are cavities that form in the underlying bone as the cartilage wears away. They can often be seen on x-ray.

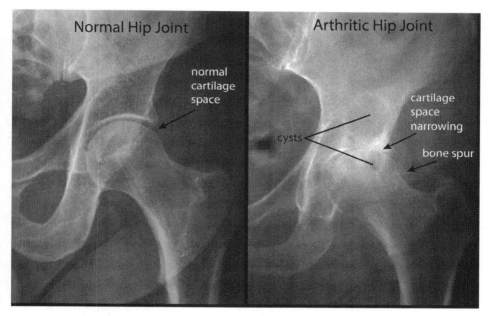

**Figure 2-3**: A normal hip x-ray compared to the arthritic hip x-ray. Note the cartilage space narrowing, bone spur, and large cysts in the arthritic hip.

## Common Misconceptions about Arthritis

Some people think arthritis is a material that forms in the hip. Arthritis is a medical condition, not a substance. You cannot scrape away, remove, or clean out inflammation and cartilage wear. It is less like the tartar that builds up on your teeth than it is like the wear on your car tires in areas where the tread is gone.

Perhaps the confusion is because when we look at an x-ray, we can see bone spurs (osteophytes) that form in response to arthritis. However, these bone spurs are just a feature or sign of arthritis and not the arthritis itself. Removal of this feature does not cure the disease.

Regarding arthritis features, let's discuss two other features that often present with arthritis (although not always). One feature is *pain*. Arthritis-related pain is complicated. For reasons that the medical community does not fully understand, arthritis does not always result in pain. In addition, the severity of arthritis as seen on an x-ray is not directly proportional to the amount of pain you may experience. In other words, we cannot tell how much pain you are having by looking at your x-ray. Some patients with mild arthritis may have severe pain, while others with severe arthritis may not have pain at all.

A second common feature of hip arthritis is *stiffness*. Sometimes the hip joint becomes so stiff that simple activities such as putting on socks and using the bathroom are difficult.

## Types of Hip Arthritis

There are three major types of hip arthritis. Each type has a unique underlying cause but produces a similar painful condition.

### Osteoarthritis

*Osteoarthritis* is by far the most common type. It is called "wear and tear" arthritis because it often has no identifiable cause and is more prevalent with age. *Osteoarthritis* is commonly confused with *osteoporosis*; however, they are not the same. *Osteoporosis* is a problem within the structure of a bone that results in decreased bone density, which then causes bones to fracture easily.

### Inflammatory arthritis

*Inflammatory arthritis* describes a group of diseases where excess inflammation occurs in the joints for unknown reasons, and cartilage wear follows.

---

### Do I need an MRI?

Most patients with hip arthritis on x-ray don't need an MRI. An MRI is only useful when the diagnosis is not clear AFTER an x-ray. In most cases, once the diagnosis is clear on x-ray, the MRI will not provide additional information that changes treatment options and it is usually not required for surgical planning.

---

*Rheumatoid arthritis* is the most common type of inflammatory arthritis. This is an *autoimmune* disorder, where the body's immune system is overactive and works against joint surfaces to break down otherwise healthy cartilage and bone.

Most people with inflammatory arthritis have seen a rheumatologist and are on special medications to treat their systemic condition. This book does not cover treatments for inflammatory arthritis.

## Post-traumatic arthritis

The third is *post-traumatic arthritis*. This occurs when a trauma such as a fracture occurs within the joint surface leading to permanent damage. When the cartilage sustains significant damage, it may do well for a period; however, over the course of months or years, worsening arthritis develops. Treatments are the same as for osteoarthritis.

## What Causes Osteoarthritis?

This question comes up frequently. It is easier to understand why cartilage wear occurs with inflammatory and post-traumatic arthritis. However, osteoarthritis is complex and *multifactorial*, which means that there are several factors contributing to it. There are *inherent* (things you can't change) and *modifiable* (things you can change) risk factors for the development of osteoarthritis (Table 2-1):

**Table 2-1:** Inherent and modifiable risk factors for osteoarthritis

| Inherent Risk Factors | Modifiable |
|:---:|:---:|
| Genetic makeup | Excess body mass |
| Gender | Sport/occupation stresses |
| Age | |
| Minor injury | |
| Luck | |

## Inherent Risk Factors – things you cannot change

- Genetic makeup: Your genes play a large role in osteoarthritis, but their exact role is not fully understood. It is not as simple as skin color or height, which can often be predicted based on your parents. Multiple genes play a role, and the interactions and expression of those genes are under current investigation.

- Gender: Osteoarthritis is more common and more severe in women than men for reasons we don't fully understand.

- Age: There is a clear correlation with age and prevalence of osteoarthritis.

- Injury: When a patient has a prior major injury such as a fracture within the hip joint or a ligament injury, we classify subsequent arthritis as post-traumatic. Patients may not recall a time long ago when they had a minor twisting injury or impact to their hip that hurt for a few days and resolved without ever seeing a doctor. We believe that some of these seemingly minor injuries can result in osteoarthritis later in life.

- Luck: Because there are so many potential causes of osteoarthritis and much of this we still do not understand, we say that luck plays a role.

## Modifiable Risk Factors—things you can change

- Excess body mass: Excess body weight can be a sensitive subject, but it is clearly linked to osteoarthritis. Obesity has reached pandemic status worldwide. Body mass affects hip arthritis in two ways. The first is intuitive: increased weight (or load) on cartilage surfaces increases the rate of wear. The second is less intuitive (and maybe more important): excess fat tissue secretes molecules in the body that increase inflammation and are thought to cause cartilage surfaces to break down. When these two mechanisms are working together, they cause the cartilage in your hips to wear at a rate higher than they would if you were at your ideal body weight. See "Calculation of Body Mass Index" below to figure out your ideal body weight.

- Sport and occupation stress: It may seem intuitive that more weight-bearing activities and stress on the hip joint would cause more wear. This is the common historical teaching of medical providers. Research has not proven this to be definitively true. Running, for example, is considered one of the biggest stressors on the hip joint, yet several studies have shown that runners do not have an increased risk of hip arthritis. There is also a theory that exercise strengthens bones and joints and therefore provides a protective effect against cartilage wear, which may counteract wear. Here is what I tell my patients: avoid running, sports, and activities that cause hip pain because if it's causing pain, it's probably causing damage; but if you can run marathons without pain in your hips, it's probably fine to continue.

## Calculation of Body Mass Index

Search the Internet for "body mass index calculator." Several will come up, and any will do the job. Enter your height and weight when prompted. Calculate your *body mass index* (BMI). Once you have calculated this, compare your BMI to the numbers below as published by the Centers for Disease Control:

Underweight <18.5
Healthy Range 18.5 – 24.9
Overweight 25.0 – 29.9
Obese ≥30.0

Obese Class I: 30 – 34.9
Obese Class II: 35 – 39.9
Obese Class III: ≥40 (also called "extreme" or "severe" obesity)

If your BMI is >30, you should strongly consider weight loss. If your BMI is >35, then you have a serious health condition that needs immediate attention. If your BMI is over forty, you should not be considering any elective surgical procedure until you have lost weight. This is a general guideline and may not apply to muscular individuals who are lean.

## Chapter 2 Review

- Arthritis = joint inflammation + cartilage wear.

- Arthritis is not a substance in your hip, it is a condition.

- Bone spurs are a result of arthritis and a sign we see on x-ray. They are not the cause of pain and are not the underlying problem.

- There are three main types of arthritis:
    1. Osteoarthritis
    2. Inflammatory arthritis
    3. Post-traumatic arthritis

- The cause of osteoarthritis is multifactorial, with many factors that you cannot control.

- Body mass index is important in determining your risk for arthritis and your risk for overall health problems.

- Arthritis encompasses a spectrum of diseases; symptoms can range from mild discomfort to severe and debilitating pain.

Chapter Three

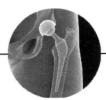

# Characteristics of Hip Osteoarthritis

## *Is it Really Hip Pain?*

I commonly see patients in my practice who believe they have a "hip" problem, and it turns out that the problem is not coming from the hip joint at all. Several other conditions mimic hip arthritis. In this chapter, we will not cover them all, and I am not asking you to diagnose your own problem, but it is important that you gain an understanding of the typical hip arthritis symptoms before pursuing treatment. If your symptoms don't match the characteristics listed in this chapter, you should question whether the hip joint is the cause.

## Location of Pain

The location of pain in the region of the hip is one of the best clues to help us identify the underlying cause. When I ask patients to point to their hip joint, they often identify the rounded area on their side near the belt line that includes the buttocks, the upper part of the pelvis, and the lower back. The actual location of the hip joint is lower and more toward the front of the pelvis than most people imagine. The location of the hip joint is shown in Figure 3-1.

Hip problems most commonly cause pain in the area we describe as the *groin* or the *inguinal crease*. When you are in a seated position, this is the diagonal crease formed by the top of your thigh and your lower abdomen.

The second most common area for pain is on the *lateral* side (lateral means 'away from the midline') of the hip. Patients with hip arthritis often grab the region around the front and side of their hip joint as the location of pain as shown in Figure 3-2. The buttock and front of

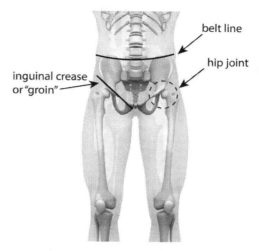

**Figure 3-1:** The location of the hip joint is shown. Note that the joint is well below the belt line. We refer to pain in this area as *groin pain*.

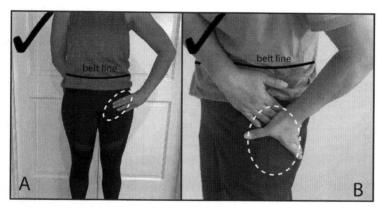

**Figure 3-2:** The two most common locations of pain from hip arthritis are A) the groin and B) the lateral side of the hip joint. Both are well below the belt line.

the thigh are the third most common areas for pain. On occasion, the knee can be painful from hip arthritis. This is a phenomenon we call *referred pain*.

If your pain is at or above the belt line, in your lower back, or the upper buttock region, the hip joint is not likely to be the cause. This is not to say that your hip region doesn't hurt, but that the *ball and socket joint* is not the cause. Figure 3-3 shows anatomic regions where the hip joint is commonly misidentified.

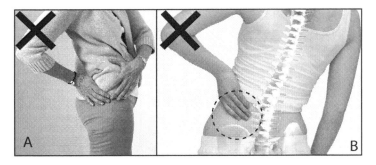

**Figure 3-3:** Patients often misidentify these regions as their hip joint. A) shows pain near the top of the pelvis, which is several inches above the actual hip joint. B) shows pain in the lower back.

## Timing of Pain

Pain from hip osteoarthritis is typically worse during or after activity and improved by rest. The afternoon or evening are usually worse than the morning. Sometimes the pain can persist during sleep at night. It is uncommon for the pain to be worse in the middle of the night than at bedtime because rest typically improves symptoms. Back problems, on the other hand, often produce pain in the hip region or down the leg that is worse at night. Pain tends to wax and wane with hip osteoarthritis – some days may be better than others.

## Types of Pain

Pain and stiffness are the two most common symptoms of hip osteoarthritis. Pain comes in many forms. Hip arthritis pain is often described as sharp, dull, or throbbing. Some patients experience a grinding or popping sensation. Hip osteoarthritis **never causes numbness or tingling** in the buttock, thigh, down the leg, or in the foot. Pain described as "burning" or "electrical" that radiates down the leg is usually coming from nerves and not the hip joint.

## Leg Lengths

Most people are not completely symmetric when it comes to leg lengths. We all have minor asymmetries. Leg length can be a complex subject that is affected by the curvature of your spine, the tilt of your pelvis, and the length of bones in your legs.

Some patients with severe hip arthritis who have worn away all the cartilage and some of the bone in the hip will notice that leg is shorter than the other side. This causes the pelvis to tilt when standing and a correlation between hip arthritis and low back pain has been reported.

## The Progression and Severity of Hip Arthritis

The natural history of hip arthritis, regardless of the type or cause, involves progression over time. Symptoms including pain, inflammation, ability exercise, and walking distance tend to worsen. Progression is often in a variable *stepwise* fashion, meaning it doesn't increase at a constant rate, but gets better, then worse, then better, then worse, etc.

Figure 3-4 shows an example of the stepwise progression of pain over time. Note the areas labeled "flare". It is common for patients to show up at a doctor's office with a bout of severe pain in a hip that has been only mildly symptomatic in the past, only to find that x-rays show the *chronic* condition of arthritis that may have been there for months or years. This is understandably puzzling to many patients but is a common feature we see almost daily. The periods of flare tend to last days or weeks, but almost always improve, especially utilizing some of the treatments listed in the chapters that follow.

The condition of arthritis encompasses a spectrum of symptoms where some patients may not be able to run but can perform all other activities pain-free. Other patients may have trouble standing, walking, or sleeping at night. On the severe end, symptoms can be debilitating and require a walker or wheelchair.

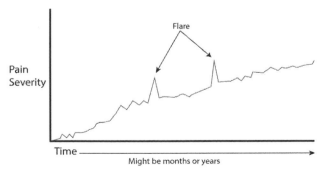

**Figure 3-4:** An example of the stepwise and variable progression of arthritis symptoms over time. The severity of pain over time will be different for every hip. Note the areas of worsening and improvement, with severe worsening known as "flare".

## Chapter 3 Review

- What many people call "hip pain" is not coming from the hip joint at all.

- Pain at or above the belt line or in the lower back is not likely coming from the hip joint.

- The hip joint is located in the groin region, and this is the most common location for arthritis pain to present.

- Arthritis pain is typically worse with activity and better with rest.

- Hip arthritis never causes numbness, tingling, or other nerve symptoms.

- A "flare" of arthritis is a dramatic acute worsening of symptoms that lasts from days to weeks but usually improves.

Chapter Four

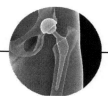

# Alternatives to Hip Replacement Surgery

### *The Kitchen Sink*

You've seen a medical provider, had an examination and x-rays, and have been told that you have hip arthritis. Now what? This chapter introduces an important concept.

For patients with moderate or severe arthritis, we currently do not have the technology to give you your previously "invincible hip" back. Anyone who promises otherwise is not giving you accurate information. We can treat symptoms, and we can replace your hip, but we cannot regrow cartilage or reverse cartilage wear. All non-surgical treatments focus on treating symptoms (mostly pain). Living an active life is most definitely achievable if you have been diagnosed with hip arthritis. The answer likely lies in this or the following chapter.

> **Important Note:** This chapter describes non-operative treatments relevant to hip *osteoarthritis* and *post-traumatic arthritis*. Inflammatory arthritis has different treatment options that should be discussed with your primary care provider or a rheumatologist.

## The Kitchen Sink

I am a strong proponent of exhausting all non-operative options prior to taking on major surgery. When you avoid surgery you also avoid all the risks that come with it. Hip replacement is major surgery and has risks that will be covered in Chapter 6.

But first, let's talk about potentially avoiding surgery by throwing the proverbial kitchen sink at the hip. In this chapter, we will outline my recommended treatment options, list some common treatments that are unproven, and also discuss some treatments to avoid. For a more in-depth discussion of each treatment, please check our companion book *Non-Surgical Treatment Options for Hip Osteoarthritis.*

## Your Primary Care Provider

Your general health is the foundation from which all abnormal conditions arise. By managing your overall health, you are managing your hip arthritis. To do this effectively, you should have an established *primary care provider* (PCP). This is an easy, no-risk recommendation for every adult. If you don't have one, find one. This could be a doctor, nurse practitioner, or physician assistant. Medical specialties that serve in the primary care provider role for adults include family practice, internal medicine, geriatrics, and in some cases gynecology/obstetrics. PCPs are a wonderful, caring group of medical providers who have a broad range of knowledge. If you develop a relationship with one, they get to know you and your medical history, which increases the quality of care. Most of the treatments in this chapter are offered by PCPs, and they will help you find the best specialist if your condition requires more specialized care.

## Scientific Evidence

In medicine, treatment recommendations are based on opinions and evidence. The scientific evidence that supports or refutes treatments is often mixed and is constantly evolving. As an orthopedic surgeon, I put a lot of trust in the American Academy of Orthopaedic Surgeons (AAOS) and their guidelines for the treatment of orthopedic conditions. The guidelines are developed by workgroups of smart, diverse, and invested surgeons and researchers who are committed to letting evidence guide treatment decisions.

The AAOS guidelines for Management of Osteoarthritis of the Hip came out in 2017.[1] The American College of Rheumatology also has guidelines that I've taken into consideration in this chapter.[2] I've blended my interpretation of these two guidelines with medical literature that has been published since 2017 and my own patient experiences to form opinions printed here. While science is paramount, there is still some art to medicine. Every surgeon's opinion and experience differ.

**<u>Recommended Non-Surgical Treatments</u>** – These include options that either have quality scientific research behind them or, in a few cases, are backed by limited science but are used widely or trusted by most surgeons. Most healthy patients can use these but always check with your medical practitioners to be sure.

| | **<u>Cautions / Risks</u>** |
|---|---|
| **Weight loss:** No treatment in this book or elsewhere has the same potential to decrease hip pain, slow the progression of arthritis, and improve your overall health like weight loss. This is *a strong* recommendation for anyone with a body mass index over thirty. See "More on Weight Loss" for more information. | *Almost no risk + high reward* |
| **Low-impact exercise**: Twenty to sixty minutes of low-impact, moderate-intensity exercise is recommended at least three days per week. Low impact exercises are those that don't put jarring or sudden forces on the hip. **Land-based** low-impact activities include outdoor or indoor cycling, elliptical trainer, rowing, cross-country skiing, and strength-based yoga. **Water-based** (pool) low impact exercises including swimming, water aerobics, water walking, water jogging, or using water weights in the pool. You may have to work to find exercises that fit your needs. | *Discuss with your doctor whether this is safe.* |

| | Cautions / Risks |
|---|---|
| **Mental health maintenance**: Mental health is linked to pain and disability. We all need to monitor our mental health. Discuss concerns with your doctor and consider an ongoing mental health maintenance program such as meditation and mindfulness exercises. See the Appendix for suggestions on books. | *Almost no risk + high reward* |
| **Physical therapy (PT):** Strengthening and stretching exercises are proven to decrease hip pain in the presence of arthritis. Technique is important for muscular strengthening. I recommend finding a coach in the form of a therapist. Even one or two visits will help guide your program. | *Avoid exercises that cause pain.* |
| **Heat and cold therapy**: These are time-tested albeit typically short-term pain relievers for osteoarthritis. You can see what works best for you, but I suggest heat before and ice after exercise or activity. A shower, bath, hot tub, or heating pad can be used for heat. Ice packs or a commercially available ice machine can be used for cold therapy. Twenty minutes up to three times per day is a reasonable start. See Chapter 8 for recommendations on ice machines. | *Use caution when putting ice or heating pads directly on the skin.* |
| **Cortisone injections:** These are also called *steroid* or *corticosteroid* injections. Cortisone a staple treatment for hip arthritis pain. Most patients get some pain relief, though results vary. Relief can range from only a few days to a few months. There are surprisingly few high-quality scientiifc | *Small risk of infection, theoretical risk of cartilage toxicity that has not been shown clinically, avoid within ninety days of knee surgery Few patients experience a "steroid* |

| | Cautions / Risks |
|---|---|
| studies looking at efficacy, but they are so commonly given that most surgeons consider them safe and effective. Avoid cortisone injections more often than every three months, and never get one within ninety days of surgery. Diabetics should be aware of a temporary spike in blood sugars from these injections. | *flare" with an increase in pain for 1–2 days after injection.* |
| **Non-steroidal anti-inflammatory medications (NSAIDs)**: NSAIDs are the primary oral medication recommended for the treatment of hip arthritis pain. They work by decreasing inflammation and pain in affected joints. Over the counter **ibuprofen** (Advil® or Motrin®) and **naproxen** (Aleve®) are the best options for most patients. There are prescription NSAIDs that are more potent but have additional risks. The lowest effective dose should be used, and intermittent use is preferred over daily use. | **Check with your primary care doctor on these.** *Use with caution if you have a history of stomach ulcers, heartburn, bleeding disorders, blood thinner use, kidney disease, high blood pressure, heart conditions, or stroke.* |
| **Acetaminophen (Tylenol®)**: Acetaminophen is a safe medication in most patients. It is generally preferred over NSAIDs if it is effective, but some patients don't see much benefit. Acetaminophen is a great option for those who can't take NSAIDs. | *Do not take with alcohol or if you have a history of liver disease. Never exceed the recommended dosages.* |
| **Cane, crutches, walker, wheelchair:** Generally, patients don't want to use these devices unless other options have failed. If you have concerns about balance or falling, go to this as a first-line option. | *Low risk but read instructions and warnings on the package for these.* |

**More on Weight Loss**

Weight loss can be life changing for anyone who is overweight, with or without knee pain. In order to accomplish something that is life changing, you will have to make significant changes in life. "How?" you may ask. That question is the basis of a weight loss industry worth over $70 Billion in the United States alone. Studies show that **diet is far more important than exercise when it comes to losing weight**. You must commit to a diet and use exercise as an adjunct to see progress. There is no single program that works for everyone. It doesn't matter if you count calories, weigh your food, avoid carbohydrates, start a new exercise program, join a gym, buy a book, take on one of the so-called "fad" diets. Take the following steps now if you think you are overweight:

1. Calculate your body mass index (see Chapter 2)
2. Discuss options with your medical practitioners. Some diets are healthier than others.
3. Find a support group. Tell your medical providers, family, and friends what your plan is and ask them to hold you accountable. This is not easy, and you will need support.
4. Commit to a plan. Expect it to require persistent work and time. It will not be easy, but you also don't have to be perfect. You just need to make lasting changes that over time will result in weight loss.
5. **YOU** can do this!

**Unproven Non-Surgical Treatments** – This section contains treatments that have been studied by the scientific community, might have some benefit, and seem safe overall, but lack sufficient evidence to support routine use.

**Massage therapy:** Most people love a good massage. However, there is no scientific data to prove its effectiveness for hip arthritis pain beyond temporary relief. If you can afford the cost, it may be worth trying, especially if other options are not available or effective.

## Cautions / Risks

*Consider cost versus benefit.*

| | |
|---|---|
| **Topical therapies:** Lotions, gels, and ointments that are rubbed into the hip have shown some benefit for arthritis pain. These are typically partial and temporary pain relievers. They make the first-line list because they are safe, cheap, and easily accessible, but be aware that studies show unimpressive results. Most are over-the-counter. **Capsaicin cream** is probably the best over-the-counter option but must be used for 1–2 weeks to see a difference. Next are **salicylate rubs** (Bengay® and Aspercreme®) and finally **counterirritants** (Icy Hot® and Biofreeze®). Prescription NSAIDs are available in topical formulations and have some scientific evidence behind their effectiveness. Discuss this with your doctor. | *Low risk but read instructions and warnings on the package for these.* |
| **Platelet-rich plasma (PRP) injections:** These injections use concentrated products derived from a patient's own blood. They are injected into the hip joint with the idea that they can reduce pain. They do not regrow cartilage or slow the process of arthritis. The scientific research is mixed but may be reasonable to consider if you have mild or moderate arthritis. Consider the cost as your insurance will not pay for this. | *Not for severe arthritis; some risk of infection; some patients have increased pain for a short period after injections; weigh the cost against modest expected benefit.* |
| **Hyaluronic acid injections**: These are also known as *viscosupplementation* injections, lubrication injections, or rooster comb injections because many pharma- | *Not for severe arthritis; some risk of infection; insurance will not pay for hyaluronic* |

| | **Cautions / Risks** |
|---|---|
| ceutical companies make them from hyaluronic acid extracted from rooster combs. Hyaluronic acid is a substance naturally present in the hip joint that is proposed to lubricate and cushion the joint. Considerable research has gone into these injections and the sum of that research shows unimpressive results. I only recommend these for select patients with arthritis on the milder end of the spectrum. I do not recommend them for severe hip arthritis. | *acid injections for the hip joint (unlike the knee where insurance often covers them.)* |
| **Acupuncture:** Traditional Chinese medicine treatments such as acupuncture have been around for thousands of years. I like the idea and the safety profile of this treatment, but the scientific evidence for treatment of arthritis pain is scarce. | *Consider cost versus benefit.* |

**Non-Surgical Options to Avoid** – Treatments on this list have studies showing that they are not effective, have limited evidence showing they are effective, need more research, and/or impose unjustifiable risk or cost to patients.

**Stem cell injections**: I'm asked about stem cell injections regularly. I strongly recommend against them. So far, the advertising and hype about stem cell injections for arthritis have surpassed science. A myriad of problems exists with the research, nomenclature, false advertising, and overstatement of stem cell therapeutic capabilities for arthritis. According to the American Association of Hip and Knee Surgeons (AAHKS) and the American Academy of Orthopaedic Surgeons (AAOS), "There is no data to support the idea that stem cells can sense the environment into which they are injected and repair damaged tissue."[3] Both organizations recommend against stem cell injections. The FDA has issued warnings about these injections and

clinics have been fined for false advertising. Despite the great promise of stem cell treatments in medicine, hip arthritis is not ready for
prime time. Do not spend your money on them until we have better
research and safer formulations.

**Opioid pain medications:** I have an even stronger recommendation against the use of opioid medications to treat arthritis pain
than for stem cell injections. Commonly prescribed opioids include
oxycodone (Percocet® or Oxycontin®), hydrocodone (Norco® or
Vicodin®), morphine (MS Contin®), hydromorphone (Dilaudid®),
and tramadol (Ultram®). We are dealing with an opioid crisis in the
United States. No country uses and abuses opiates more than we do.
No medication I prescribe has more side effects or higher addictive
potential. The AAHKS also has a position statement against opiate
use for arthritis which sums up my personal opinion: "It is our position that the use of opioids for the treatment of osteoarthritis of the
hip and knee should be avoided and reserved only for exceptional
circumstances."[4] Don't take opioids for arthritis pain. If you are on
these medications, ask your doctor to help wean you off them.

**High-impact exercise:** While there is a debate among medical providers as to whether high-impact activities cause arthritis, most
practitioners agree that people with hip arthritis or hip pain should
avoid such activities. You can increase your risks of cartilage wear
and worsening symptoms by engaging in high-impact exercise.

**Therapeutic ultrasound:** Ultrasound is useful as an imaging technique but far less useful as a therapeutic measure for hip arthritis.

**Cupping therapy**: When the most decorated Olympian of all-time
competed in 2016 with cupping marks all over his body, it invigo-
rated this alternative treatment. It lacks quality scientific support for
its use for the condition of hip arthritis.

**Laser therapy**: Laser therapy is another alternative treatment that
is not ready for mainstream acceptance based on a lack of quality
research.

**Prolotherapy**: Prolotherapy uses a sugar solution that's injected into the hip and shows promise as a future treatment option. I feel that this injection is not worth the unknown risks without more research data.

**Supplements:** The use of supplements to treat arthritis pain is a controversial subject. As a society, we love our supplements. Most people like the fact that they are a more "natural" version of medications, though I dispute this idea. Supplements are concentrated chemical formulations just like medications. Any substance ingested for an intended chemical effect has the potential for side effects and adverse reactions. A 2015 study showed that an estimated 23,000 people visit the emergency room every year for adverse events related to supplements, including those taken for pain and arthritis.[5]

There are certainly some legitimate uses of vitamins and supplements for health, but if you are looking for hip arthritis treatments backed by science, look elsewhere. There is no high-quality scientific research showing that supplements alleviate osteoarthritis symptoms. This includes **glucosamine** and **chondroitin**. The American Academy of Orthopaedic Surgeons states a strong recommendation against the use of either of these commonly used supplements[6]. There is a lack of scientific evidence for efficacy against hip arthritis other commonly used supplements including: turmeric, rose hip, avocado soybean unsaponifiables (ASU), methylsulfonylmethane (MSM), willow bark, and omega-3 fatty acids. The other, potentially bigger, issue with supplements is that they are unregulated. You truly do not know exactly what you are taking, how much you are taking, and how safe it is despite what it says on the bottle.

Cannabidiol, also known as CBD, deserves special mention as a supplement because of its growing popularity and availability. This is a non-psychoactive derivative of marijuana plants. There is no shortage of anecdotal support behind CBD and its psychoactive sibling, tetrahydrocannabinol (THC). Results of quality research into the pain-relieving and anti-inflammatory effects of CBD has been called "underwhelming" and "insufficient" by pain management researchers.[7] Animal studies and small clinical trials in humans show some potential, but CBD should be considered at best a second-line treatment, and it is not the cure-all that is sometimes advertised. It is not without side effects and risks, and is primarily sold as an unregulated supplement, which means you can't be sure the product label is accurate. Read this Harvard Health blog listed in the Appendix for a fair review of CBD.[8]

## What About Hip Arthroscopy?

Patients sometimes as if a "clean out" scope would be helpful for their arthritic hip. The scientific evidence is clear that hip arthroscopy is not helpful in the presence of arthritis. Remember, arthritis is a condition and not a substance. You can't just "clean out" worn cartilage and expect a good outcome. This will only expose more bone and leave behind more worn cartilage.

## Chapter 4 Review

- Non-operative treatments for hip arthritis cannot replace or repair cartilage.

- Try non-operative treatments before moving on to a hip replacement. If you find a safe and effective non-operative treatment, go with it.

- Non-operative treatments have varying degrees of scientific evidence to support their use. Rely primarily on science rather than anecdotes when choosing your treatments.

- Some of the most effective treatments are lifestyle changes: weight loss, aerobic exercise, strengthening exercises, and mental-health awareness.

- Science does not support many of the trendy treatments for hip arthritis including acupuncture, cupping, and supplements.

- Stem cell injections currently have many problems in their formulations, research, advertising, and cost. There is not enough scientific evidence to justify the risk and cost of these injections.

- Do not take opioid pain medications, except in very rare circumstances.

- Supplements, including glucosamine and chondroitin, have no proven benefit for hip arthritis pain or protection of cartilage.

- CBD may have some benefits for pain and inflammation of joints but needs more research into efficacy and safety. It is currently an unregulated supplement.

- Hip arthroscopy is not a viable treatment option for hip arthritis.

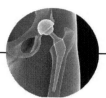

Chapter Five

# Understanding Hip Replacement Surgery

## *The Definitive Solution for Hip Arthritis*

Your hip hurts. You've already thrown the kitchen sink of non-operative treatments at it, but your pain persists. Hip arthritis symptoms are different for every patient and they range from mild to severe. If your pain is mild, it might be an annoyance that you can live with. Many patients with severe hip pain lose their active lifestyle. Some gain weight, become depressed, and their overall health suffers. Luckily, we have an excellent solution.

In the previous chapter, we established that once cartilage is worn away, we do not have a reliable non-operative method to replace or repair that cartilage. The only time-tested option to replace worn cartilage is a hip replacement surgery. Let's talk about what this means and how a hip replacement solves the problem of hip arthritis definitively.

## A Brief History of Hip Replacements

The medical term for hip replacement is hip *arthroplasty*. Remember from Chapter 2 that "*arthron*" means joint. The medical term "*plasty*" means to mold or shape to restore form and function. These two words combine to form artho-plasty which is the term commonly used by medical providers. When we replace both the worn ball and the socket within the hip joint to restore form and function this is called a *total hip arthroplasty.*

The earliest documented attempts at hip replacement were around 1891. Surgeons used materials such as ivory, plaster of Paris, skin, fat, and pig bladders to replace the worn bone and cartilage within the hip joint without much success. During the early 1900s and into the 1950s, other materials were used to replace worn bone and cartilage including glass and stainless steel. The stainless-steel version had some success, but the results were not ready for the masses.

Sir John Charnley, a British orthopedic surgeon, is credited with developing the modern hip replacement in the 1960s. The implants he designed used a combination of metal, plastic, and bone cement to replace worn cartilage and bone. In the 1970s, Charles Anderson Engh, an innovative surgeon at the Anderson Orthopaedic Clinic in Virginia, developed porous hip implants that allow the bone to grow into them without bone cement.

Historically, hip replacements took several hours to perform, and patients remained in the hospital for days or weeks at a time. With advancements in anesthesia, surgical techniques, and post-operative care, hip replacements have changed dramatically since Charnley and Engh's pioneering days, even though we still employ some of their design principles.

## Hip Replacements Today

Total hip replacement is now considered one of the most successful procedures the of last sixty years and has been dubbed "the operation of the century."[9] It remains the gold standard of treatments for severe hip arthritis.

Approximately 400,000 hip replacements are performed annually in the United States. That number is expected to double before 2035 because of population growth and aging baby boomers. The mean age for a hip replacement is sixty-five years; however, any adult with arthritis might qualify.

Hip replacements are safely performed in small community hospitals, outpatient surgery centers, and in large medical centers. The life expectancy of a modern hip replacement exceeds twenty years.

The surgery typically takes one to two hours, and the length of stay in a medical facility ranges from hours to a few days.

## What Exactly Happens in a Total Hip Replacement?

Recall that when both sides of hip the hip joint have worn cartilage, the ball and socket joint are rough (Figure 5-1). This causes pain, inflammation, and in some cases a grinding sensation in the hip joint.

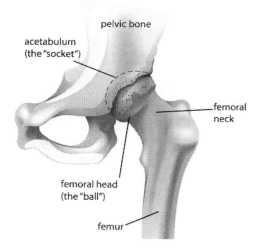

**Figure 5-1:** Review of what the arthritic hip looks like with worn joint surfaces.

To relieve the pain and inflammation, we replace the worn ball and socket with prosthetic *components* (which are the parts used in the hip replacement.) Figure 5-2 shows the components used to replace bone and cartilage.

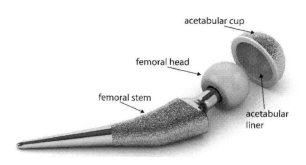

**Figure 5-2**: Components (parts) used in hip replacement surgery.

Let's see a step-by-step illustration of how these components are inserted into the hip joint during a total hip replacement (Figure 5-3). First, a skin incision is made and the muscles and other soft tissues around the hip are pushed aside to access the joint. The location of the incision depends on the *surgical approach* which is covered in more detail below. The typical steps then follow:

1.  A cut is made across the *femoral neck* and the femoral head (the "ball") is removed from the *acetabulum* (the "hip socket").

2.  The acetabulum is prepared for the new hemispherical metal *cup* using a device called a *reamer.*

3.  The porous titanium cup with a *polyethylene* (plastic) liner is then pressed tightly into the space created by the reamer. The cup size is measured to fit each patient. It fits securely, and with time, bone grows into the porous metal. Sometimes screws are inserted through the cup to help hold it in place.

4.  The *femoral canal* is then prepared to accept the porous *femoral stem*. The native canal is a hollow cylinder with soft marrow inside.

5.  The femoral stem is inserted into the femoral canal. The size of the stem depends on the size of the canal and is fit to each patient at the time of surgery. This is press-fit tightly into place, and, like the cup, bone grows into the stem over time. In some cases, the stem is held in place with bone cement.

6.  A ball is placed on top of the femoral stem, and the ball is inserted into the socket, which recreates the hip joint. After all of the components are securely in place, the incision is closed with sutures, staples, and/or skin glue. Final x-rays are usually taken in the operating room or the recovery room.

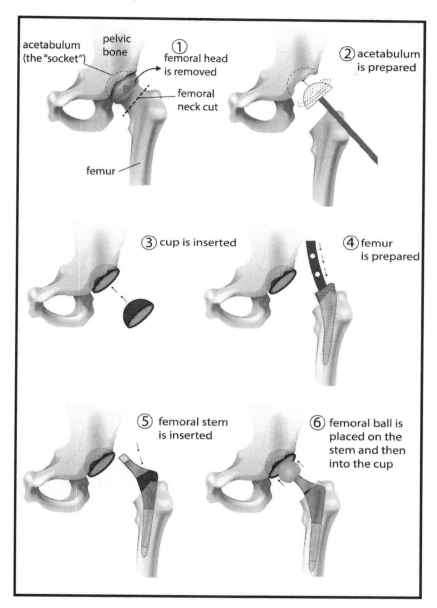

**Figure 5-3**: Steps in a hip replacement surgery. See the accompanying text for a description.

## Total Hip Replacement Surgery Variables

Some variables depend purely on surgeon preference. There is a lot of debate (and no clear answer) as to whether certain variables lead to better outcomes. I suggest you go with the options that your surgeon prefers and <u>do not try to dictate these variables</u>. Asking your surgeon to change their preferred methods to something you read about is more likely to hurt your outcome than help it. For the curious patient, the variables for hip replacementare listed below.

## Manufacturer/Model

I have experience using components from several joint replacement manufacturers. I am not aware of any conclusive evidence that one brand or model is superior to others. Asking surgeons which company is superior is akin to asking a crowd of people if Ford or Chevrolet is superior. You will get a lot of strong opinions, but nobody knows for sure.

Even within a single manufacturer, there are different model choices. The models differ mainly in the design of the femoral stem. Models have different geometries, lengths, and coatings (Figure 5-4). If you are curious, it's fair to ask your surgeon about their rationale for choosing an implant and what his overall experience has been. Most surgeons do not receive money from implant manufacturers. Kickbacks are illegal and closely monitored. The surgeons that do receive funding from implant companies are consultants for design, teaching, or research.

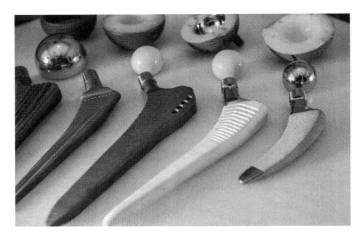

**Figure 5-4**: Examples of different hip component shapes and sizes.

## Use of Bone Cement

In the United States, the majority of surgeons do not use bone cement for hip replacements. Most use the porous-coated variety that allows bone to grow into them. In some parts of the United States and in much of Europe, the femoral stem is cemented into place. There are abundant studies showing excellent results with both cemented and uncemented constructs.

## Bearing Surfaces

*Bearing surfaces* are the two parts that rub together in the joint: the femoral head and the acetabular liner (the ball and the socket). The femoral head is most commonly metal (cobalt chrome) or ceramic. The majority of acetabular liners are *polyethylene* (plastic), and in rare circumstances are metal or ceramic. In the early 2000s, a metal head was sometimes placed on a metal liner, but over time, this combination of surfaces caused metal ions to shed into the surrounding hip tissues and the bloodstream. This combination is called *metal-on-metal* and is rarely used today because of high failure rates and some product recalls. I use and recommend a ceramic head on a polyethylene liner for all hip replacement patients because I believe this construct is least susceptible to complications and has a proven track record for longevity.

# Hip Resurfacing

A variant of hip replacement is resurfacing. This option uses the same type of cup as a total hip replacement, but the side of the femur the head is shaved down and a metal surface is capped with a metal piece over the end. (Figure 5-5) Touted advantages include an easier revision in the future (if needed), and a lower rate of dislocation (when the ball comes out of the socket). Disadvantages include potential fracture of the femoral neck after surgery, and this construct uses a large metal head on a metal liner. Most surgeons are concerned about the metal-on-metal problems described above, and I believe the risks associated with the shedding of metal ions outweigh the potential advantages. Some surgeons still use hip resurfacings, so their opinion differs from mine.

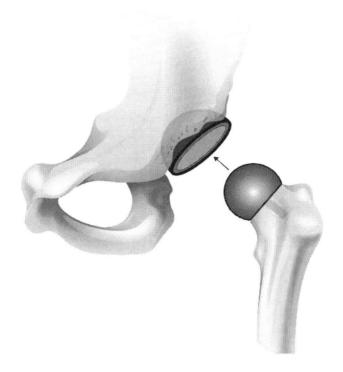

**Figure 5-5:** Hip resurfacing is similar to total hip replacement, but there is no stem going down the femoral canal.

## Surgical Approaches

The term *surgical approach* describes how the surgeon gets into and exposes the hip joint. The approach begins with the incision location (Figure 5-6). The different approaches are like different doors all leading to the same room. Commonly used approaches are posterior (back door), lateral (side door), anterolateral (a door midway between the front and side), anterior (front door) and the two-incision approach (working through two doors or windows simultaneously).

Some approaches are dubbed *minimally invasive,* but no clear definition exists for what constitutes minimally invasive versus a standard approach. I consider an approach minimally invasive if it avoids splitting individual muscles and uses a skin incision that is shorter than about six inches (15 cm).

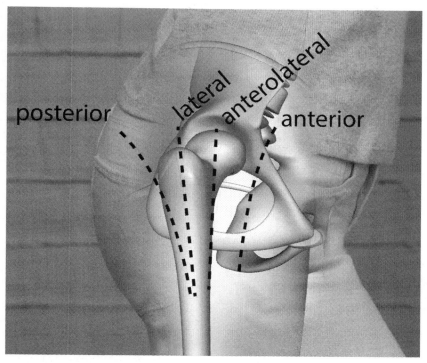

**Figure 5-6:** Incision locations for four commonly used surgical approaches to the hip joint.

Now the inevitable question: which approach is best? The answer: the one your surgeon is most comfortable with. There is no one approach that has been proven via clinical studies to be better than the others for long-term outcomes. Surgeons feel strongly about the approach they choose, and each approach has documented pros and cons. Choose your surgeon first (see Chapter 7) and go with the approach your surgeon feels is best for you.

I personally favor the direct anterior approach (going in through the front of the hip) and I use a specialized table (also optional) in the operating room to help expose the hip, shown in Figure 5-7A. This particular approach has been growing in popularity over the last ten years and is one of the most common today. Other approaches such as the commonly used posterior approach use a standard table and the patient is placed on their side for the surgery as shown in Figure 5-7B. The direct anterior approach is considered minimally invasive because we work between muscular planes and not through them. Some studies show patients recover faster using this technique. I've used other common approaches, and, in my hands, the anterior approach provides the most consistent results. Compared to when I used the posterior approach, I make a smaller incision, I give patients less postoperative restrictions, and patients take fewer pain medications. This approach also facilitates the use of x-ray in the operating room which provides quality control throughout the procedure.

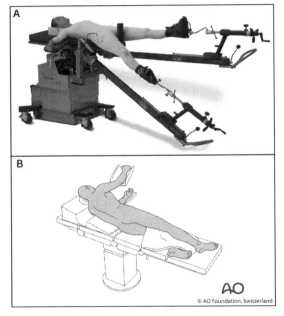

**Figure 5-7**: A) A specialized table – the Hana® table – assists in hip joint exposure with the anterior approach. B) Other approaches may place the patient on their side to expose the joint. (Images used with permission, see Appendix for image credits and copyrights.)

## Optional Hip Replacement Technology

Technology is an important part of improving outcomes in hip replacement. However, more surgeons adopt technology when clinical studies prove that technology does one or more of the following:

- decreases complications
- increases patient satisfaction
- enhances short or long-term success rates
- aids in recovery

- decreases the overall cost of the procedure

Computer-assisted and robotic surgery have become the standard of care in some fields of surgery. They are gaining ground in joint replacement surgery, but studies do not show better functional outcomes. Additional downsides are increased costs and longer surgery times.

- **Computer-Assisted Surgical Navigation**: This technology uses computers and imaging to assist the surgeon in placing the components in an optimal position. Computer-assisted surgical navigation is a promising technology that will continue to grow, although studies do not demonstrate a significant advantage in terms of outcomes. I use a form of this technology because it helps me achieve more consistent results, but I don't feel it is critical.

- **Robotic Surgery**: This is another technology that will continue to grow. It's hard to imagine that in twenty years we all will not be doing robotic and/or computer-assisted hip replacements. Today's technology has some touted advantages, but again, its outcomes are not significantly better than obtained from an experienced surgeon using standard instruments. Robotic surgery is expensive, and I know some surgeons who use it for knee replacements but feel it's less useful for hips. Someday it may have more clear advantages.

## Same-Day Discharge Hip Replacements

Surgical equipment, surgical techniques, anesthesia techniques, medications, and other processes around hip replacement have advanced to the point where patients can go home the day of the surgery. Surgery can be performed in a stand-alone surgery center or in a hospital with same-day discharge.

Multiple studies have proven that same-day discharge is safe, and most patients are satisfied with this option. The advantages of being discharged on the same day include the comfort of staying in your own bed and having more friends and family around to help. Being at home from the beginning will also empower you to take care of yourself. One main disadvantage is that your healthcare team will not be available immediately should any complications or concerns arise.

Although same-day discharge is gaining popularity, some surgeons and hospitals won't allow it. Other locations may not have the proper systems in place, or there may be insurance restrictions that preclude going home the same day.

The key here is that the proper systems must be in place, and patients must be properly selected for same-day discharge. Only the healthiest, most motivated, knowledgeable, and mobile patients should be offered this option.

## Need Both Hips Replaced?

I often see patients who have severe arthritis in both hips and are ready to have both replaced. The question arises, how do we approach this?

*Staged bilateral* hip replacements is the term that describes replacing both hips on different days. The length of time between the first and second varies by patient and by surgeon. My preference is to wait a minimum of six to eight weeks before operating on the second hip – enough time to get over the initial healing phase for the first hip and prepare for the second. The overall risk of staged bilateral procedures is probably lower (some studies refute this), but patients need to plan for two surgeries. If you choose this option, do the hip that hurts more in the first procedure, even if it has less arthritis on x-ray.

*Simultaneous bilateral* replacements are done on the same day, in the same surgical setting. The surgery takes roughly twice as long, and the patient takes on one recovery period instead of two. It is important to understand that this option is significantly more painful (some would say twice as painful). Some studies suggest that this option has more risks. I do not offer this option to patients unless they meet strict health criteria and understand the pain will be increased. Some surgeons do not do it at all because of the perceived risk.

This is a decision you should discuss with your surgeon and those caring for you. For most patients, the staged bilateral procedure is a better option.

## Chapter 5 Review

- Hip replacements have evolved over the last century into one of the most successful and most common procedures performed today.

- A hip replacement utilizes a combination of metal, ceramic, polyethylene (plastic), and sometimes bone cement to replace the worn bone and cartilage surfaces of the hip joint.

- Hip resurfacing is an option to a total hip replacement but has the significant disadvantage of using a metal head on a metal liner – a construct that has proven to have many issues.

- Surgeons have different preferences for the surgical approach. Studies have not shown a difference between different surgical approaches for long-term outcomes.

- Technology such as surgical navigation and robotics are helpful to some surgeons, but studies have not shown a significant improvement in clinical outcomes with these technologies.

- Some joint replacement centers are allowing patients to go home the day of surgery. Studies have shown this is safe as long as protocols are in place and patients are carefully selected.

- If both hips need to be replaced, you may have the choice to do them both on the same day or on two days separated by a healing period. For most patients, doing the hips six to eight weeks apart is a better choice.

Chapter Six

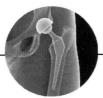

# Results of Hip Replacement Surgery
## *The +90 Rule*

We make medical decisions based on whether the proposed benefits justify the costs. Costs may be in the form of money, time, or risks. Either consciously or subconsciously, we are constantly undertaking this risk/benefit analysis for when to take a pill, get an injection, or have surgery.

Each patient that undergoes hip replacement surgery has a different risk profile. I suggest you be deliberate about evaluating your personal risks and potential benefits of surgery. This analysis will require the help of your medical practitioners, and this chapter will get you started in thinking about some important factors.

## Who Qualifies for Hip Replacement Surgery?

In my practice, patients must meet five criteria to move forward with hip replacement.

1. **Moderate or severe arthritis** must be present on x-ray. Mild arthritis is not good enough to qualify. In addition, MRI scans are less useful because they often exaggerate the amount of cartilage wear.

2. **Daily, life-limiting pain symptoms** must be present. It is not worth the time, effort, and risk if the pain is mild or occasional.

3. **Non-operative measures have failed**. I want patients to have tried something else – anything else. I have a hard time jumping into surgery without at least attempting less invasive measures.

4. **Patients are healthy enough for surgery**. Most people meet this criterion, but there are some patients in which the risk of surgery exceeds the benefit. We often involve primary care providers and other medical specialists to help make this decision.

5. **Patients must understand the procedure.** By reading this book, you are covering this one. Patients and their support teams (family or friends) must understand the procedure, the risks, the benefits, and expected outcomes.

---

### Too Young or Too Old?

Notice that age is not listed in the criteria for who qualifies for hip replacement. If you are thirty-five, have severe arthritis on x-ray, and meet the other four criteria, then it might be the right operation for you. Surgeons might hesitate with younger patients only because the patients may outlive their replaced hip, requiring a revision surgery. If you are ninety-five and meet all the criteria, then it also might be a good operation. The ninety-five-year-old must understand that medical risks of surgery are high. The thirty-five-year-old and the ninety-five-year-old have different risk factors based on age, but they both might be good candidates for the surgery.

---

## Benefits of Hip Replacement Surgery

Hip replacement is primarily a pain-relieving procedure. The secondary benefit is improved quality of life. Patients achieve these benefits the vast majority of the time. It is common for hip replacement patients to say after surgery, "I wish I would have done that sooner."

To say that we are aiming to decrease pain and improve quality of life is not very specific. You will notice that I did not say, "Eliminate pain and give you a perfect hip." Hip replacement is an excellent operation with high success rates, but it's not perfect. Let us talk about what that means and how much improvement in pain and quality of life you should expect.

We cannot give you back the *invincible hip* discussed in Chapter 2. We are talking about replacing human tissue with an artificial hip made of metal and plastic. MOST patients can expect the following:

1. **Pain relief**: Some patients achieve 100 percent pain relief with hip replacement. Others, though significantly improved, will not be 100 percent pain-free. Expect some minor or occasional pains even after hip replacement.

2. **Significant improvement in function**: Function has to do with how you move through each day of your life. A painful hip literally affects every step. Hip replacement should allow you to walk, put on your clothes, drive, and go to the store more comfortably and more efficiently. Stiffness in the joint is a common complaint prior to surgery. Patients often have difficulty putting on shoes and socks. This procedure improves the range of motion in most patients.

3. **Return to low-impact activities you previously enjoyed**: If your hip is the limiting factor for activities, replacement should help you return to those you previously enjoyed. Most patients can safely walk, hike, bike, use an elliptical trainer, swim, ski groomed runs, and play golf if they enjoyed these activities before arthritis. If other medical conditions limit these activities, the hip replacement will not overcome them.

## Avoiding Misconceptions of Benefits

Let's bring some clarity to what hip replacement is NOT likely to do. The items on this list are important to understand, and most have to do with symptoms away from and not related to an arthritic hip joint.

1. **Body mass index**: Many patients believe that hip replacement will be the key to weight loss because they can exercise. It turns out that MOST patients do not lose weight after hip replacement. Some gain weight because diet is more important than exercise for weight loss, and hip replacement does not directly influence eating habits.

2. **Balance**: Balance worsens with age, and it is often related to systems outside of the leg and hip joint. I mention this because some patients are disappointed that they still have balance difficulties after a successful hip replacement.

3.  **Back pain**: Back pain is sometimes connected to a hip prob-
    lem. Often, it is a separate issue. Most patients I see with low
    back pain and hip arthritis continue to have back pain after hip
    replacement.

4.  **Running, jogging, or other high-intensity sports**: Hip replace-
    ments are not made for impact activities. Activities that involve
    sprinting, cutting, pivoting, and jumping should be avoided. I
    have some patients who continue to jog after having their hip
    replaced and some compete in endurance sports at a high level.
    The hard surfaces in the hip replacement can be unforgiving, and
    anyone taking on impact sports should be aware that these ac-
    tivities have the potential to affect the longevity of the replaced
    joint.

5.  **Fibromyalgia or other chronic pains**: Surgery will not change
    any pain generated systemically outside of the hip joint.

6.  **Numbness and tingling**: Numbness or tingling in your legs,
    feet, or toes are not likely to be caused by an arthritic hip, so a
    hip replacement will not change these symptoms.

## Risks of Hip Replacement Surgery

If hip replacement surgery were always 100 percent successful, risk-
free, and lasted forever, surgeons would recommend this procedure
for even mild arthritis. However, every surgery carries risks.

There are three types of risks associated with hip replacement.

1.  **Surgical risks**: These are risks associated with the surgery itself.
    Luckily, complications during surgery are uncommon.

2.  **Medical risks**: These are risks that happen after surgery. They
    are indirectly related to the surgery but caused either by the
    stress of surgery on the body or medications given with sur-
    gery. Medical complications occur more frequently than surgical
    complications.

3.  **Pain and functional risks**: These risks have to do with your
    outcome. Even with a perfect surgery and no medical complica-
    tions, pain and function after surgery can be unpredictable.

## Surgical Risks

These risks are directly related to the surgery itself and/or anesthesia. During surgery, there is a small risk of bleeding, fracture of the bones, or inadvertent injury to nerves, vessels, tendons, and ligaments. Delayed surgery-related complications include infection, loosening of the prosthetic components, joint instability, and wear of prosthetic components. Anesthesia complications should also be considered but are very uncommon with modern anesthetic techniques.

Available studies have variable numbers to define the percentage of patients that have surgical complications, so I'm going to give some estimates that are admittedly rough approximations based on available scientific data. My goal is to give you an idea of the rarity of the complications above. For example, an injury to the major nerve that runs behind the hip joint occurs in 1-2 percent of patients. Injury to large blood vessels around the hip occurs less than 0.3 percent of the time. The numbers in Table 6-1 show estimates of risks based on rough averages from multiple studies.

A few potential complications require special mention. Infection, when it occurs in the prosthetic hip joint, is a devastating complication. Luckily it occurs in less than 1 out of every 100 patients. *Dislocation*, where the ball pops out of the socket after surgery, is an uncommon but scary complication because it requires a visit to the emergency room to put the ball back where it belongs. Studies are quite varied on the overall incidence, so I estimate up to 5 percent of patients have this complication after their first hip replacement. I have seen a lower incidence of dislocations with the anterior approach, but that finding is not universal and is not substantiated by scientific studies. Since we are fitting joint replacement parts tightly into the bones of the pelvis and femur, fracture of those bones during surgery is a risk. The overall incidence is around 1 percent.

## Medical Risks

Anytime we put the human body through the stress of anesthesia and a major surgery such as hip replacement, we must account for risks away from the surgery site. Not only is the surgery itself a risk, but the medications we give to help with surgery and recovery have potential side effects.

Medical complications are one of the major considerations of hip replacement surgery and depend on a patient's underlying health conditions. Examples of medical risks include blood clots in the legs or lungs or complications with the heart, lungs, liver, and kidneys. If these occur, most happen in the first few days after surgery, but the risk may extend for weeks or longer in some cases. Minor medical complications such as nausea, constipation, and dizziness are common. We are constantly watching for these and generally have answers for them. Major complications such as kidney failure, heart attack, and stroke are less common, and I estimate that significant medical complications occur less than 5 percent of the time in patients who are properly selected and medically screened before surgery.

## Venous Thromboembolism (VTE)

*Venous thromboembolism* (VTE) is the medical term for blood clots that occur in the veins of the body. This risk deserves its own discussion because it can happen in any patient and has the potential to be serious. The two primary places blood clots occur are in the legs (called *deep vein thrombosis* or *DVT*) and in the lungs (called *pulmonary embolism* or *PE*). Treatments that attempt to avoid a complication are termed *prophylaxis*. Without VTE prophylaxis, some studies quote rates of higher than 50 percent for DVT or PE. With proper prophylaxis, that rate drops to around 1-2 percent.

We think about VTE for two reasons. First, DVT can cause pain and swelling in the legs. Secondly, if a PE forms in the lungs, it can be life-threatening. Prophylactic measures that help avoid VTE include activating your leg muscles after surgery, using special compression devices on the legs, and using a blood-thinning medication. This topic will be discussed further in later chapters when we discuss recovery after surgery.

**Table 6-1:** Risks with hip replacements (approximate)

| Risk | Approximate Incidence (varies between studies) |
|---|---|
| Numbness around the incision site | >50% |
| Noticeable leg length differences | 5% |
| Unexplained pain | <5% |
| Major medical complications | <5% |
| Dislocation | <5% |
| Plastic liner wears out | <5% |
| Loosening of components | 3-5% |
| Neurologic or vascular injury | <2% |
| Symptomatic DVT or PE | 1-2% |
| Fracture during surgery | 1% |
| Infection | <1% |

## Pain and Functional Risks

Even when your surgery goes perfectly and there are no medical complications, and even when you follow your postoperative rehabilitation instructions to the letter, there is a risk that pain and function will not meet your expectations. This is one of the most unpredictable parts of hip replacement and is frustrating for the patient and the surgeon when it occurs.

## Successful Surgery and the 90+ Rule

There is debate in the orthopedic community about how to gauge the success of a surgery. Do we judge it by complications, patient satisfaction with the process, or patient satisfaction with the outcome? The answers to these questions are not clear.

Researchers have developed questionnaires to determine patient satisfaction, and, in my opinion, these are the best current measure of success. If you can answer "Yes" to the question, "Are you satisfied with your hip replacement?" then it was the right decision. The answer to this question considers complications, pain, and function, and is different from the questions, "Is your hip perfect?" or "Did you have any complications?"

Here is where we end up with what I call "The 90+ Rule". My interpretation of available studies and my own experience with hip replacement show at least a 90 percent satisfaction rate. In other words, 90 percent or more of patients undergoing hip replacement would do the surgery again or would recommend the surgery to a friend or relative. It turns out that who is satisfied and who is not depends heavily on patient characteristics, some of which we can change and some we cannot.

## Modifiable Risk Factors

We can influence patient satisfaction and outcomes after surgery by modifying factors within our control.

Let's go through the modifiable factors, one at a time:

- **Body mass index (BMI)**: An elevated BMI increases your risk of surgery complications. The higher your BMI, the more at risk you will be for infections, wound drainage, blood clots, complications during surgery, medical complications, pain levels after surgery, and dissatisfaction after surgery. Higher body mass index not only increases the amount of soft tissue that has to heal around the incision, it affects metabolic pathways in the body that play a role in healing.

- **Tobacco or nicotine use**: Nicotine causes constriction of blood vessels, impairs healing, and increases infection rates. In addition, smokers tend to have worse lung function and more pain after hip replacement. It does not matter if you smoke cigarettes, use a vaping device, chew tobacco, or use cigars – they all have nicotine. Tobacco has thousands of other chemicals that are harmful to overall health and healing after surgery.

- **Drug abuse:** Illicit drugs impair function, healing, compliance, social interactions, sleep, and cause many other negative aspects that affect surgical outcomes.

- **Alcohol use:** Consuming more than two alcoholic beverages per day in the month preceding surgery can increase the risks of complications. The liver is critical for healing after surgery, and alcohol impairs liver function with increased use.

- **Blood sugar control:** This one is for diabetic patients. Patients with diabetes have been shown to have twice as many postoperative complications in some studies. There is a lot of debate and conflicting studies on whether *hemoglobin A1c* predicts complications after surgery. What almost everyone agrees on is that good blood sugar control before and after surgery is critical.

- **Preoperative opioid pain medications**: As recommended in Chapter Four, you should not be on opioid pain medications for arthritis pain. Studies show three important findings on opioid use prior to surgery. First, if you are on these medications prior to surgery, pain after surgery may be more difficult to control. Secondly, patients on opioids have more medical complications after surgery and lower satisfaction rates. Finally, if you come off opioids prior to surgery, the risks mentioned reverse; meaning pain control improves, risks go down, and satisfaction with the outcome increases.

- **Amount of hip arthritis on x-ray**: Studies have shown that patients with milder arthritis on x-ray are more likely to have pain after surgery.

- **Dentition**: Dental problems, especially when they involve cavities and infection, put patients at risk for hip joint infection after surgery.

- **Nutritional status**: Protein malnutrition is seen primarily in three groups: elderly, the extremely thin, and (paradoxically) in the obese. Overweight patients may be nutritionally deficient because many foods that promote fat formation are also nutritionally deficient (think sugars and other carbohydrates). Nutrition is most often measured by *albumin* which is a protein measured in the blood. Several good studies have shown that low albumin levels correlate with complications.

- **Anemia:** *Anemia* is low red blood cell counts or decreased ability for red blood cells to carry oxygen via the carrier *hemoglobin*. If you have anemia going into surgery, and you lose more blood during surgery, this condition can present complications.

## Non-Modifiable Risk Factors

Other risk factors are not modifiable, meaning we can't make changes to improve the risk profile.

- **Age:** We've previously established that there is no magical cutoff number that determines when a patient should and should not have a hip replacement. I find the overall health and functional status of individual patients to be more important predictors of success, so age should never be a standalone determinant of fitness for surgery. When we look at the population as a whole, age is a factor for complications that seems to increase more significantly after seventy-five.

- **Diabetes:** An argument can be made that diabetes is a modifiable risk factor for some patients who are obese. For others, it is not something that can change. Either way, it increases risks of complications, especially for patients who require insulin.

- **Heart or lung disease**: There is a broad spectrum of severity of heart and lung diseases, but your surgeon should take note of any such condition in and discuss the risks before surgery.

- **Liver disease:** The liver is a critical regulator of physiology after surgery. Patients with active liver diseases such as cirrhosis, hepatitis, or other impaired functions are at increased risk for complications.

- **Kidney disease**: Kidney function is measured by a blood test, and those with lower function are at higher risk for complications. Another concern is that patients with impaired kidney function have fewer pain medication options around the time of surgery.

- **Prior surgery**: Studies show that patients with any prior hip surgery have a slightly increased risk of infection with hip replacement surgery.

- **Blood disorders**: Patients who have a propensity to bleed or form clots excessively have an increased risk of complications. It is important to let your surgeon know if you have one of these disorders or take any blood-thinning medications.

- **Immune deficiency:** Having an impaired immune system increases the risk of infection and decreases the body's ability to heal after surgery. Examples of diseases that can cause such impairment include HIV/AIDS and drug-induced immune deficiencies.

- **Rheumatologic disease**: Rheumatologic diseases alter the body's immune system functions, and some medications taken for these diseases do the same. Again, an impaired immune system can lead to infection and other risks.

- **Fibromyalgia or chronic pain syndrome**: These poorly understood disorders cause pain. The result after surgery is typically more pain and lower satisfaction with the result.

- **Mental health disorders**: Patients with anxiety and depression are often less satisfied with the result of hip replacement. Both disorders are linked to pain. Proper treatment can help decrease this risk.

- **Multiple medication allergies or sensitivities:** Patients with multiple reported medication allergies tend to have worse outcomes with surgery. The cause of this is not clear, but it seems that some patients are more sensitive to medications than others, and the risk of having an adverse reaction to a medication or surgery goes up when more allergies are reported. Allergies might also limit our ability to give preferred medications during and after surgery.

## Chapter 6 Review

- Establishing the benefits and expectations after hip replacement is an important preoperative task.

- Three types of risks are associated with hip replacement: surgical, medical, and pain/functional. It is important that both the patient and the medical teams understand these risks.

- Approximately 90 percent of all patients who have hip replacement are satisfied with the outcome. Some causes of dissatisfaction are hard to predict.

- Modifiable risk factors are those that we can change before surgery. We should make every effort to change them to maximize the outcome.

- Non-modifiable risk factors cannot be changed and understanding them is important to assess the overall risk of the procedure.

Chapter Seven

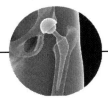

# Choosing Your Team
## *The Right Support*

This is your surgery, your body, and you have to live with the outcome. You need to take charge of who helps you achieve a successful hip replacement. Don't rely on other people to do this for you. It's been my experience that patients who take responsibility for their own health and medical decisions have the best outcomes. Let's discuss how to select and recruit people who are going to give you the best support and outcome.

## Your Surgeon

Choosing your surgeon is not always easy. We all want the best available to do our hip replacements. There are no universal guides, formulas, or rating systems that will lead you to the best surgeons.

Before I go into some recommendations on how you might choose a surgeon, let me first endorse my colleagues and my profession. Orthopedic surgery residencies are among the most competitive to get into out of medical school. No matter who you choose, he or she was likely at the top of their medical school class and has completed nine or more years of formal medical education and training after college. He or she has passed tests and been the subject of close scrutiny throughout his or her career.

Just like any other profession, however, there is a spectrum of training, knowledge, talent, effort, and surgical skill. It is also important to point out that because of my background, training, and experience, I may value different factors when choosing a surgeon than other practitioners in this profession.

## Choose and Trust

No single factor on the list below would cause me to rule in or rule out a surgeon from performing a quality hip replacement. Use the best information you have available to you, choose your surgeon, and, finally, trust his or her methods and techniques. Certainly, you should ask questions about things that don't make sense and advocate for yourself, but also trust his or her experience. Hip replacement surgery is a combination of science and art, and to do his or her best work, your surgeon needs some freedom to practice his or her way.

## The Surgeon versus the Auto Mechanic

Orthopedic surgery has some similarities to fixing cars. Both require knowledge and manual dexterity. Both are professions where repetition and training make a difference. There are talented and knowledgeable mechanics who can fix just about anything with a combustion engine. Mechanics who are more specialized might just fix one brand or model. On average, the specialized mechanic will fix a specialized car more efficiently and accurately than the general mechanic will.

Like the auto industry, orthopedic surgery has become more sub-specialized than ever. Some general orthopedists dabble in a little bit of everything, while specialists focus on a small number of body parts. There is more to excellent surgeons than training, repetitions, and specialization. Innate talent, for example, is also important, and not measurable. If we are talking averages, however, it would be hard to argue against a more experienced, more specialized surgeon.

## Specific Surgeon Factors to Evaluate

Each of the items listed is one part of the equation that maximizes your chances of a good outcome. None of these factors is a stand-alone dealmaker or deal-breaker when choosing your surgeon.

1. **Number of hip replacements per year**: If all else is equal, several studies have shown that the more hip replacements a surgeon performs per year the better a patient's chance of a good outcome from a procedure performed by this surgeon. There is

no well-established guideline or cutoff for the number of surgeries per year a surgeon should perform. In the absence of universally accepted definitions, I am going to give my subjective and potentially biased interpretation of the available studies. I would think twice about a surgeon who does fewer than thirty hip replacements per year. This is fewer than three per month and is *low volume*. Available studies show a clear correlation between lower volume, higher complications, and need for revision surgery. As we move closer to seventy-five hip replacements per year, my confidence starts to grow because the repetition and experience are better. Above 150 per year, a substantial portion of the surgeon's practice is dedicated to hip replacements. Most surgeons do not perform more than 300 per year, but the highest volume surgeons might do 400 or more hip replacements per year.

2.   **Fellowship training**: Anyone who is licensed and credentialed to perform hip replacements in the United States has completed medical school and at least a five-year orthopedic residency training program. After residency, surgeons can go directly into practice, or they can choose to do an additional year of subspecialty training called a *fellowship*. Adult hip and knee reconstruction fellowships typically require twelve months of supervised training in primary, revision, and complex hip replacement surgeries. These are the true sub-specialists of hip replacement. The extra training is meaningful.

3.   **ABOS certification**: It is surprising to some that orthopedic surgeons are not required to be board-certified to practice, though most are. The largest certifying body is the American Board of Orthopaedic Surgery (ABOS). To earn ABOS certification, surgeons must pass a written exam, be in practice for two years, and then take an oral exam. Every ten years, this certification must be updated. If your surgeon is board-certified, he or she has passed written and oral exams, and has practiced for at least two years. This combination of experience and knowledge demonstration is helpful. For more information on board certification or to check if a potential surgeon is board-certified, the

ABOS has a useful look-up site: **https://mycertifiedorthopae-dicsurgeon.org**

4.  **Years in practice:** Years in practice can function as a bell curve with respect to surgical skills. Early in their careers, surgeons have less experience but more recent training. They also tend not to have age-related physical limitations. At the back end of a surgical career, experience peaks. However, surgeons are less likely to take on new techniques late in their careers and aging often leads to a decline in sensory and motor skills. Let us estimate that a typical surgical career is around thirty years. I've always felt that the middle twenty years of that career are probably a surgeon's best. This phase of the career balances experience, skill, drive, receptiveness to innovation, and physical dexterity.

5.  **Professional reputation:** If you know someone who works in a local orthopedic clinic, hospital, or especially an operating room, this might be a good resource. Clinic staff will know if a surgeon takes responsibility for patients. Operating room staff will have some sense of skill and efficiency. There is one word of caution here. Surgeons are often judged in the work setting by personality and temperament. On many occasions, I have met beloved, caring, and personable surgeons with comparatively weak surgical skills, and I know surgeons with disagreeable temperaments or poor interpersonal skills who are outstanding technicians.

6.  **Reputation within a community:** Community reputation is worthwhile, although it is a weak indicator of a surgeon's skill. Community reputation is influenced by many factors that have little to do with surgery and some that do. If a surgeon is well regarded in a community, it certainly does not hurt; just be aware that it is not everything.

## Surgeon Factors That Probably Don't Matter

1.  **Medical school and residency institution**: I've met many doctors since I started medical school in 2001, and I have never

drawn a clear correlation between the name of a school and the knowledge or skill of its graduates. The same is true for residency training. Some of the more famous Ivy League schools look good on a resume, but I know surgeons who went to little-known medical schools whose surgical skills exceed those of Ivy Leaguers. If your surgeon went to an accredited medical school and completed an accredited orthopedic residency program, the location or name of that institution should not be used as a pro or con in surgeon choice.

2.   **Position or job title:** It has been my overall experience that if a surgeon is labeled Chief, Director, Chairperson, or maintains some other title in their department or hospital, it should not play a role in choosing him or her. These job titles are certainly earned and should be respected, but the reasons they are assigned to that role may or might not have to do with surgical skill or quality of patient care.

3.   **Practice type or location**: A quality hip replacement can be performed through a large academic institution, a private hospital, an HMO, or at a small community hospital. All have potential advantages and disadvantages and this factor alone should play no role in surgeon choice. The only caveat here is that the volume of joint replacements at a hospital might correlate with the quality of outcomes. This is discussed further below.

4.   **Use of robots, computers, or other technology**: As was discussed in Chapter 5, we are not at a point where anyone can say definitively that the use of robots, computer navigation, or other advanced technologies consistently provide better surgical outcomes. If your surgeon uses advanced technologies and feels that he or she personally can do a better job with the technology, then I am all for it. If your surgeon believes that using conventional hip instrumentation and techniques gives him or her the best chance at a quality outcome, then it's easy to support this approach as well. These are topics that surgeons and medical studies debate heavily, but you should remove them from your decision.

## Location of Surgery

The type of hospital or surgery center and geographic location are not generally predictive of outcomes. I don't make a distinction between a hospital or a stand-alone surgery center because there are advantages to both.

However, just as surgeon expertise has some correlation with volume, the same is true for the processes and procedures in a hospital or surgery center. Nurses, surgical techs, and other support staff might have more familiarity with joint replacement patients if they care for these types of patients regularly.

An argument can also be made that more personalized care occurs at a low-volume facility, but if all else is equal, studies support lower complication rates at higher volume centers.

## Physical Therapist

The therapist-patient relationship is important for surgery recovery. Patients have different preferences for style. Some want to be pushed and others want gentle care. My best advice is to start with a therapist recommended by your surgeon, family member, or friend. You might even consider booking a *prehab* (therapy before surgery) appointment to start getting familiar with your therapist and make sure it's a good fit. Establishing this relationship and expectations after surgery will benefit you both. Over the years, I have appreciated therapists who:

1. **Understand the differences between recovery after hip replacements compared to knee replacements:** I have different protocols for postoperative physical therapy after hip replacements compared to knee replacements. Long-term stiffness is a concern with knee replacements, so I have my patients start therapy right away. Hip replacements rarely, if ever, get stiff. Overdoing the early therapy after hip replacement can cause setbacks and complications, and for this reason, I recommend little to no therapy in the first six weeks after surgery in my patients. In my practice, the role of therapy comes later for strengthening and gait training.

2. **Outline your plan and set goals**: Patients appreciate knowing what is important at each phase of recovery. Experienced therapists understand your goals and limitations. They provide reassurance that you are on track and tell you when you are overdoing it. Ask for an updated plan of care at each session.

3. **Are clear about expectations and goals between appointments**: Most of your physical therapy will be done outside of therapy sessions. If you expect the therapist to do the work for you, your outcome will be compromised.

4. **Provide written reports for your surgeon**: It works best if you hand-carry these reports to your surgeon appointments. When they are faxed or mailed, the surgeon often does not see them unless they share the same electronic medical record system.

## Joint Replacement Coach

A joint replacement coach is someone who is close to you to and invested in your outcome; typically, a family member or close friend. A good coach will learn the educational materials with you before surgery, attend your preoperative classes and other appointments, and be there to care for you when you get home. Give him or her a copy of this book or other educational materials provided by your surgeon.

Unforeseeable incidents often come up that we cannot predict. When you have the support of a close companion, it is less stressful to make decisions on how to handle these unplanned events. It is also helpful to have a second set of eyes and ears because the volume of information you receive during this journey is substantial. Every surgeon has instructions specific to their postoperative care. Medications are usually given on a schedule and it can be helpful to have someone monitoring that. Finally, when the going gets rough, and it might, you need someone to reassure you that you will get better.

## Help at Home

The amount of help you will need at home is patient-specific. At a minimum, I suggest that someone is available full-time for the first

seventy-two hours after you arrive home from the hospital or surgery center. Once you have two to three days to gauge how much
help you will need, you can reassess how much he or she needs to be
there. Choose someone who is close to you. This person should be
able to handle bathroom and bathing duties should the need arise.
Your helper can also be your coach.

Those helping at your home should also be able to help you
with meals. We will discuss meals further in Chapter 8. Most patients
can stand and walk around the house but standing for extended periods to prepare meals might be difficult.

## Your Driver

Assign someone to drive you to the hospital or surgery center on
the day of surgery, back to your home, and around town to various
post-surgery appointments. We will talk more about when you will
be able to drive again in Chapter 11.

## Chapter 7 Review

- Choosing your support team is an important part of the
  surgical process.

- Choosing the best surgeon for you is challenging. Some
  surgeon attributes to look for include advanced training, board certification, experience, and reputation.

- Your physical therapist is part of your recovery team,
  and you should consider a *prehab* appointment to establish a relationship.

- From your pool of close family and friends, you should
  select a joint replacement coach, those who can help at
  home, and a driver. These can be the same or different
  people.

#### Chapter Eight

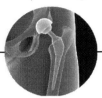

# Preparing for Surgery
## *Set Yourself Up for Success*

Hip replacement is not something you just show up and do. It takes preparation. This chapter maintains the theme that patients who take charge of their own health have fewer complications and higher satisfaction rates after surgery. Construct a well-conceived preoperative plan. This will help set you up for a successful outcome.

## Schedule Your Surgery

One of the first tasks is to schedule your surgery date. Hip replacement is elective surgery, meaning it can be scheduled well in advance and is rarely urgent. That is not to say that if the pain is severe, you should not move forward quickly. Remember from Chapter 2 that the natural history of hip arthritis is that it typically progresses slowly over time. From a technical standpoint, the surgery is usually not more difficult or risky if it is delayed a few months.

My advice is to undergo surgery when it works well with the rest of your life so give yourself time to complete the tasks in this chapter. I typically recommend a minimum of three to four weeks to complete these tasks. Coordinate the best time with your employer, your support team, and anyone else who will be affected by surgery.

## Mental Preparation

Preparing mentally for surgery is a recommendation that the medical community underrates. This does not mean you should perseverate about the surgery date or stress about the outcomes. My advice is the opposite. The goals of mental preparation are to increase your awareness of how you feel emotionally and give you the mindset that maximizes your ability to deal with stress after surgery.

Stress and anxiety are normal emotions that surround surgical procedures. They leave us vulnerable and are a significant deviation from our normal routines. An important first step is to accept these emotions as normal.

If you have previously diagnosed anxiety, depression, or other mental health disorders, make sure you are happy with your current treatment plan. If you don't have a prior diagnosis but have concerns, I strongly urge you to address them with your primary care provider before surgery. Anxiety and depression are extremely common and are underdiagnosed. Having the awareness to address these issues is a strength and not a weakness. There are abundant resources for diagnosis and treatment.

Even if you are happy with your current mental health, I recommend mindfulness exercises as a tool, even if you are not having surgery, but especially if you are. I have no professional expertise in this field, but I've listed resources in the Appendix by some who have that expertise.

Pain has cognitive, behavioral, and emotional components. The amount of pain you experience after surgery will be affected by your awareness of these components. You can start practicing some exercises before surgery that address pain. Dealing with the pain starts with an acknowledgment. I recommend conscious and positive self-talk with phrases such as, "This hurts, but I know it will be okay," or "It's going to be difficult for a while, but I will get back on track."

Resilience plays an important role in recovering from hip replacement. I define this as the ability to adapt to stressful and painful situations and maintain a positive attitude after surgery. Resilience can improve pain levels. Research shows cognitive behavioral therapy can boost resilience after surgery, and I suggest it even for individuals with good mental health. See an introductory resource for this in the Appendix.

## Physical Preparation

Ideally, patients who qualify for hip replacements would have already tried formal physical therapy to treat arthritis pain. Physical therapy is beneficial even if it does not solve the problem completely. One advantage of physical therapy is that it helps prepare your hip for surgery.

A single appointment with a licensed therapist (ideally the therapist who will help you during your postoperative rehab) is a great idea. It will give you the chance to connect with your therapist and receive advanced coaching on exercise techniques.

A low-impact exercise program is also important for overall health, as long as it does not cause significant pain. Do not start a new exercise routine just before the surgery.

Eating a healthy diet is also part of your physical preparation for surgery. Do not start any new diets just before surgery but follow healthy eating guidelines. Before and after surgery it is advisable to eat a diet high in vegetables and fruit, with some protein in the form of meats, seafood, or meat substitutes.

## Home Preparation

The two primary goals of preparing the home before surgery are to avoid falls and make sure the items you need are conveniently accessible. Declutter your home to avoid falls. Remove items that are a tripping or slipping hazard, including loose cords, loose rugs, toys, and small furniture. Most patients do not need to install special handrails around the house, but I recommend this if you think you might need them for an extended period after surgery.

A common question is whether you should move your bedroom to the ground floor. Most patients can safely navigate a flight of stairs after surgery. You should receive instructions before discharge from the medical facility on how to go up and down stairs. If you have significant weakness or inability to go up and down stairs prior to surgery, then moving your bedroom to the first floor is not a bad idea.

Preparing or purchasing frozen meals prior to surgery is helpful. You will want quick and easy meals for the first one to two weeks.

Plan a pre-surgery shopping trip to stock up, not only on food supplies but on household supplies such as toilet paper, paper towels, bathroom supplies, and other commonly used household goods.

Do your laundry just before surgery so that you have a nice stock of clean clothes. You will also want to have clean sheets on your bed when you arrive home.

## Equipment to Borrow or Purchase

I recommend a four-point walker for most patients after hip replacement. The style most patients prefer is foldable (so it can fit in the car easily), has adjustable height, and has wheels on the front (Figure 8-1). While you can put your full weight on your hip after surgery, the main purpose of the walker is to improve your balance and help you avoid falls in the early recovery period. You can purchase this from a local medical supply store or online. A quality walker should cost less than $30 on amazon.com. Search for "Folding Walker with 5-Inch Wheels".

A cane is also a good idea for most patients. A few patients go directly to the cane after surgery, but most use it when they have graduated from the walker. Two styles are shown in Figure 8-1. A single-point cane is enough for most, but some prefer a four-point cane. These are available online or at drug stores for under $20.

Putting ice on the hip is important after surgery. There are several options for this. The first is a commercially available ice machine. These consist of a cooler or basin filled with water and ice, tubing, and a cuff that wraps around the hip. Search "ice machine hip" on amazon.com and different styles and prices will result. Your surgeon or the hospital may also have them at a discounted price. Ice machines are not cheap, but most patients feel they are worth the cost because of the extensive amount of icing that occurs after surgery. The second option is specialized gel packs that can be frozen and wrapped around the hip. The third option is large frozen vegetable bags (peas tend to work well). Last, plastic bags filled with ice can be used. You'll want to purchase large freezer bags that seal for this.

There are a few other recovery aids that can be helpful for home care, including an extended shoehorn, a Sock-Aid®, and a reaching/

grabbing device. On amazon.com search for "hip replacement recovery kit" and several packages with these devices will result. A shower seat stool is convenient to have. This helps you to avoid standing for prolonged periods in the shower. Some patients find a raised toilet seat with handles convenient. Standard toilets are low to the ground and it can be difficult for some to stand independently from that position for the first few weeks after surgery. Low toilet seats present a dislocation risk for some surgical approaches. The shower seat and raised toilet seat can also be ordered online for around $30 each.

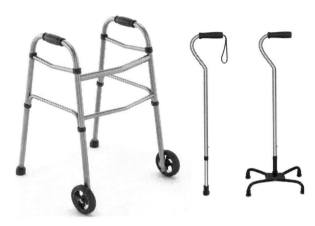

**Figure 8-1:** Assistive devices including a four-point wheeled walker, single-point cane, and four-point cane.

## Medical Optimization

Your medical team wants you to be in the best physical condition possible for surgery. You may hear the term *medical clearance* which describes seeing a medical provider (someone other than the surgeon) prior to surgery and having that provider say that you are healthy enough to proceed. Many providers don't like the term clearance because it implies that surgery is either safe or not safe. As we've discussed previously, everyone faces different risks with surgery.

You will need an appointment to evaluate your underlying medical conditions. This typically needs to be performed and documented **within thirty days of surgery.** If it is more than thirty days before surgery, you may have to repeat the exam. If you have conditions that might put you in a high-risk category for surgery, your surgeon might recommend an appointment with your primary care provider or a specialist before the thirty-day window so that you have more time to work on medical issues.

Typical options for the optimization appointment are your primary care provider or a specialized pre-op clinic. If you don't have a primary care provider, now is a great time to get one and have a full history and physical. A provider with expertise in medical conditions should discuss your history, perform an examination, and listen to your heart and lungs. Tests performed before surgery usually include at least an electrocardiogram (EKG) and some blood labs. Optional tests include a chest x-ray and urine sample. Depending on your history, your healthcare team may choose to order more extensive tests to examine your breathing or heart functions and check for anything that signals a potential risk for surgery.

You might also employ the help of specialists. If you have a history of significant heart issues, it might be worthwhile to have a discussion with your cardiologist. If you have a neurologic disorder or have had a stroke previously, your neurologist may be helpful. The same goes for lung, kidney, liver, or any other medical issues that are chronic, for which you have seen a specialist.

## Modifiable Risk Factors and Self-Optimization

Based on your history, you may have the opportunity to improve your health prior to surgery. These topics should be discussed with your primary care provider and your surgeon. Remember the modifiable risk factors we discussed in Chapter 6? These are so important that I'm intentionally repeating them here. You may have the option to work on them prior to surgery. In many cases, I even suggest a discussion with your surgeon on delaying surgery if you think you can make progress in any of these areas:

1. **Body mass index:** If your BMI is over thirty, I recommend weight loss. If it is over thirty-five, I strongly recommend weight loss. If it is over forty, I recommend you delay surgery until you've lost weight. Because there is a correlation between BMI and

complications, you can really improve your chances of a good outcome by lowering your BMI. Make sure you lose weight in a healthy manner. It is not a good idea to do a "crash diet" right before surgery as this might affect your nutritional status. Talk with your medical provider about the best options for you.

2. **Opioid use:** Opioid use prior to surgery makes postoperative pain control more difficult and decreases patient satisfaction with the surgery. Work with your prescribing provider to decrease your use, and ideally, you should have a holiday from any opioids for one month prior to surgery.

3. **Nicotine or tobacco use:** May joint replacement centers will no longer offer elective hip replacement to patients who use nicotine or tobacco products. Use surgery as a reason to quit forever. It is best to discontinue use completely at least six weeks prior to surgery. The CDC has some useful resources at www.cdc.gov/tobacco.

4. **Diabetes**: If you are diabetic, most surgeons would prefer that your hemoglobin A1c is less than eight prior to surgery. More importantly, you should closely monitor your blood sugars in the weeks leading up to surgery as well as after surgery. Check with your primary care provider if you think you need better control.

5. **Alcohol use**: If you drink regularly, consume two or fewer drinks per day for a month before surgery. It's even better if you can abstain from alcohol. Your liver function is important for recovery, and alcohol can impede your liver.

6. **Dentist**: Make sure you don't have any cavities, infections, or other dental problems prior to surgery. If you have known problems, have them treated well before surgery. I recommend a dental appointment within six months of hip replacement. If you haven't seen a dentist in that window, make an appointment for an exam and cleaning. I recommend that you don't have any dental work done within two weeks of surgery, so plan this ahead of time.

7.  **Sleep apnea**: Risk factors for sleep apnea include snoring, waking up a lot at night, being overly tired during the day, being overweight, or having a large neck circumference. If one or more of these apply to you, I suggest that you are screened for sleep apnea. Sleep apnea is a relatively common and potentially serious disorder that causes you to stop and restart breathing while sleeping. This can be a dangerous disease with surgery, especially when we add medications like opioids. If there is any question, get it checked out prior to surgery by your primary care provider.

## Reasons to Contact Your Surgeon Before Surgery

Even after you have set up your surgery date and followed every recommendation to the letter, unexpected things may happen, and some of these occurrences may make the risk of surgery unacceptable. In these unique instances, canceling or postponing your surgery might be best for your overall health.

Some examples of when to contact your surgeon or primary care provider immediately include:

- You become pregnant
- Infection of any type within seven days of surgery – even if you are on antibiotics
- New blood clot anywhere in the body
- New diagnosis of sleep apnea that's untreated
- New stroke or aneurysm
- New heart condition or a heart attack
- Difficulty breathing or shortness of breath
- Chest pain with exertion (example: when climbing up the stairs or exercising)
- Diarrhea or vomiting within three days of surgery
- Severe cold within three days of surgery
- New diagnosis of cancer

- You are drinking alcohol heavily or using illegal drugs
- New blood-thinning medications
- You have no help at home after surgery

## Chapter 8 Review

- Pick a surgery date that works for your lifestyle, family, and friends. There is no rush to undergo hip replacement.

- Preparing mentally for surgery can increase your chances of a successful outcome and decrease pain with surgery.

- Preparing physically for surgery can speed recovery and connect you to a physical therapist.

- You should have a pre-operative appointment with a medical specialist prior to surgery and undergo the process of medical optimization.

- If you have modifiable risk factors for complications, you should work to minimize or eliminate these.

- Education before surgery is critical. Kudos for reading this book! If your hospital or surgeon offers a class, take it.

- There are some good reasons to delay or cancel the surgery. Contact your surgeon if you develop a new condition that might compromise your surgery results.

Chapter Nine

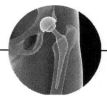

# The Day of Surgery
## *Your Day to Relax*

You read it right. Surgery day is your day to relax. For most of the hip replacement journey, it is important that you take charge and be involved in every step. This is the one day where you let go, put your faith in others, and go along for the ride. You have done your job leading up to this point, and it's time to let your chosen team take over.

If you have taken my recommendations for mental preparation, you may have some new cognitive behavioral or meditation skills to use. Regardless of your choice, try to relax and enjoy the process.

It is completely normal to be nervous. Do not apologize or worry about it. It is a natural part of this process, and there are some advantages to recognizing anxiety and accepting it as normal.

## At Home Before Surgery

The night before your surgery, try to get some good sleep. I suggest against any sleep aids unless you have cleared them with your medical providers. Avoid alcohol the night before surgery.

You should have some very clear instructions from your surgeon or the medical facility where your surgery is being performed. If you have not received these, check with your surgeon's office. These instructions might include:

- Medications to take and avoid before surgery. For example, some blood pressure medications may be taken, but some should be avoided.

- When you should have your last food or drink. This differs by facility, and there are often separate instructions for **solid foods** and **clear liquids**.
- Time of arrival for surgery. Do not be late. The operating room runs on a tight schedule and late arrival can delay other patients.
- When to shower before surgery and what type of soap to use.
- When to stop shaving your legs. Using a razor in the days leading up to surgery may increase your infection risk.
- What to wear. Dress in comfortable, loose-fitting clothes
- Don't wear makeup, perfume, cologne, aftershave, or deodorant. Some other patients are sensitive to strong scents.
- Avoid using any lotions on your skin after your last preoperative shower.
- Avoid nail polish or artificial nails because they affect the ability to read your pulse using a fingertip pulse oximeter.
- Wear glasses rather than contact lenses.
- Remove any body piercings.
- DO NOT write YES, NO, or anything else on your body to indicate the correct surgery site. This causes confusion and the site will be marked by the surgical team after arrival.
- Most hospitals and surgery centers have policies against nicotine and cannabis products, and they may jeopardize your outcome, so leave them at home. If you require a nicotine patch, let your surgeon prescribe it.

## Items to Bring with You

The following list consists of typical items that are recommended:

- Picture identification and insurance card
- A list of your current medications with dosages
- A credit card for co-pays
- Toiletries
- A change of clothes if you are staying overnight (loose-fitting pajamas, athletic shorts, and t-shirts are good)

- Undergarments
- Hearing aids, dentures, and eyeglasses
- A sleep apnea machine if you have one (CPAP or APAP)
- If you have a walker and cane, you might bring them so the therapists can adjust them to the proper height (ask first)
- An ice machine if you purchased one
- Books, tablet, laptop, and cell phone – most hospitals have Wi-Fi available. Don't forget chargers for your electronic devices.
- Flat, slip-resistant, supportive shoes

Leave these items at home unless they are specifically recommended by your surgeon or the hospital:

- Your own medications
- Cash, jewelry, and other valuables
- Contact lenses (bring eyeglasses instead)

## Arrival at the Medical Facility

Aim to arrive a bit early. This can prevent anxiety and account for things such as traffic and time to walk into the surgery center. You will typically check in at a front desk. Have your photo ID and insurance card ready. You might need to pay a co-pay at this time.

## The Preoperative Area

When it is your turn, you will be brought back to the preoperative area. This is where the medical team will begin to prepare you for surgery. You will probably be asked to take off your clothes and put on a hospital gown.

The nursing staff will ask you questions and make sure that you've followed your pre-hospital instructions. Answer their questions as accurately as possible. Have your medication list with dosages available. Make sure they are aware of any drug allergies. After they have completed the necessary paperwork, they will:

- Listen to your heart and lungs.

- Place an IV – this is typically in the arm or the hand.

- They may shave any hair around the incision site. It is important that you don't do this yourself before the surgery. They use a special sterile razor.

- They might wipe down your surgery site with some antibacterial wipes.

- You will likely receive some IV fluids before surgery.

- The anesthesiologist might order some pre-op medications for pain or to counteract the side effects of anesthesia.

- Some anesthesiologists will order a patch to be placed behind your ear to help with nausea.

- You will meet with the anesthesiologist or nurse anesthetist prior to surgery. He or she will ask more detailed questions about your medical history and your past experiences with anesthesia and will perform a brief airway exam. This is the time when the anesthesiologist has a discussion regarding what type of anesthesia to use. You should go with their recommendation. Remember, he or she does this every day and is looking out for your best interests. You will discuss the risks and benefits of different types of anesthesia and will sign a form stating that you've had this discussion. There are three common options which are all safe and effective:

- **General anesthesia**: This is still commonly used and involves putting you to sleep completely. A tube is placed either down your throat or in the back of your throat to breathe for you. Some anesthesiologists prefer this on all patients, others use it for select patients.

- **Spinal anesthetic**: This is similar to an epidural given for childbirth, except instead of leaving a catheter in place, a single injection is given around the nerves in the lower part of your back. This removes pain sensation and temporarily renders you unable to move from the waist down. You might still feel pressure but not pain below the waist. With this option, you breathe on your own, and a sedative is also given so that you are relaxed and not aware of what is happening in the operating room. Spinal anesthetic is my preference, but I leave that decision to the anesthesiologist and the patient.

- **Regional block**: Some anesthesiologists and surgeons prefer an injection around one of the major nerves in the hip or leg areas to cause numbness in the nerves below that location. This option is hospital and surgeon dependent and is often given in conjunction with a general or spinal anesthetic.

Your surgeon (or possibly an assistant) will also meet with you in the preoperative area to answer any last-minute questions and have you sign the surgery consent form. The surgeon should also put his or her initials on the surgery site as a double-check.

When all the preoperative tasks are complete, it's time to give hugs and kisses to loved ones and head back for surgery. You will see them before you know it with your new hip!

## The Operating Room (OR)

Depending on whether you receive a sedative in pre-op, you may or may not remember much of the operating room. You will be rolled into the room on a bed, and there will be several people present including one or more people from the anesthesia team, surgical assistants, an operating room nurse, and possibly sales representatives that handle surgical products used by the surgeon. It is perfectly normal to be bashful about having body parts exposed that most people don't see. We have seen it all before, and we don't think twice about it. Try not to think about it and understand that these are all medical professionals who take your privacy seriously. They are there to help you and to make you comfortable.

You will be moved to an OR bed. A urinary catheter might be placed (I rarely use one on my patients). The OR team will also get you in the correct position on the table. Don't try to help, just relax, take deep breaths, and think of your favorite place to be and who you would be with. The blood pressure cuff placed on your arm may squeeze tightly and cause some temporary discomfort. This will improve. The anesthetic given through your IV may cause a significant burn in the arm. This is expected, and before you know it, the pain will go away, and you will drift off to sleep. The next thing you know, you will be in the recovery room waking up.

The process of surgery, including anesthesia, positioning, and the surgery itself, takes anywhere from one to three hours, depending on the hospital, the complexity of the surgery, and the surgeon. The time for surgery can vary, so don't let a longer or shorter-than-anticipated surgery concern you or those waiting for you.

Before you leave the operating room, a *surgical dressing* (the bandage over the incision) will be placed. Historically a drain has been placed in the hip joint at the end of the surgery, but good studies have shown that it makes no difference, so I find that most surgeons are not using them. The surgeon will often update your family or friends immediately following the procedure.

## The Recovery Room

After the general anesthetic or sedatives have worn off, you will wake up in the recovery room. You will have a new team of nurses and nursing assistants caring for you. They are experienced in watching patients wake up and guiding them through the early phases of recovery.

With time, you'll sit up, start to take in ice or fluids, and maybe move on to some simple foods. Nausea is common, so go slow. Communicate with the recovery room staff about your pain levels as they have medications available if it's not controlled. Sometimes routine x-rays are taken in the recovery room as well. Sometimes the nurses will allow your loved ones to visit you in the recovery room after you wake up.

For patients having surgery in the hospital, the recovery room is often a temporary stop before transferring you to your overnight hospital room. Once you've met certain milestones with respect to alertness, pain levels, and vital signs, and your medical condition appears stable, you will be transferred to your hospital room.

For patients going home on the day of surgery, you will spend the remainder of your time in the recovery room. Typically, you will still have to meet the same criteria for discharge as are listed in the section entitled "Criteria for Discharge Home" in the next chapter.

## Pain Control Following Surgery

In the recovery room, you will be asked about your pain levels. There are no hard rules about how much pain you will have in the recovery room or beyond. It varies greatly from person to person. How much pain you have will depend on your own physiology, what medications you've received, whether you had a spinal anesthetic or regional block, and whether the surgeon injected pain medications around the surgery site. A general anesthetic puts you to sleep but has no effect on pain levels when you wake up.

If you received a spinal anesthetic, regional block, or medications were injected around the surgery site, you might wake up from surgery with no pain. This is normal in some patients. Other patients wake up with pain despite these measures. If you have minimal to no pain, know that with time it is likely to increase as the medication wears off, which can be anywhere from a few hours to twenty-four hours after removal of the medication.

Measuring pain is challenging because it is a subjective sensation. One of the common methods for assessing pain is called the visual analog scale. It is a scale where we ask patients to rate pain from 0 (no pain at all) to 10 (worst pain you can imagine). I find this tool modestly helpful because a 9 out of 10 pain for one patient might be a 3 out of 10 for another. Many patients will overstate their pain in order to get the message across. It is in your best interest to give your medical team an honest assessment.

One of the most important rules of hip replacement is this: **the goal is not to have zero pain.** This goal is not realistic. It can be dangerous if you hope to achieve zero pain with pain medications. **The goal is TOLERABLE pain while resting**. For most patients, this is achieving a level 4 or less out of 10 when lying in bed or sitting. Your pain is expected to increase with movement.

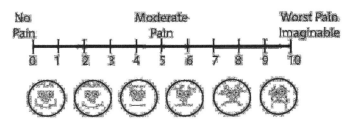

**Figure 9-1**: The visual analog scale used to identify pain after surgery.

## Chapter 9 Review

- The day of surgery is the day you get to relax and let others work.

- Anxiety is normal on the day of surgery but do your best to relax.

- There are lists of things you should and should not bring to the hospital in this chapter that are worth reviewing before the surgery.

- Arrive early and prepare to meet several people in the preoperative area as you get prepared for the operating room.

- The anesthesiologist is your best resource to discuss anesthesia options.

- A separate team will care for you in the operating room. The total time in the operating room can be from one to three hours.

- After surgery, you will spend some time in the recovery room. From there, patients who stay overnight will be moved to their overnight room.

- Pain after surgery is hard to predict. The goal for pain is never zero. Decide on what pain level is tolerable for you and communicate honestly with your care providers.

Chapter 10

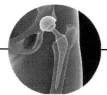

# The Hospital Stay

## *Keep it Short*

Most patients will stay at least one night in a medical facility after hip replacement. Historically, patients have stayed days or weeks in the hospital after this procedure. Over the past several years, the medical community has started to look critically at what services we are actually providing patients in the hospital, and the effect of longer stays on outcomes and complications. We have learned that as long as patients are medically stable, recovery at home has a better outcome than in a medical facility with respect to progress and outcomes. Many centers now have programs to go home on the day of surgery, which is safe for carefully selected patients. In my practice, most patients stay just one night.

Plan for the shortest stay possible. You will sleep better at home, you have more control over food and visitors, and the home provides an environment of normalcy and wellness. The sooner you get home, the faster you will take control of your own recovery.

Now, let's talk about what happens in the hospital and what it takes to get home.

## The Overnight Hospital Room

From the recovery room, you will be moved to your overnight room (also called the *ward*) once some specific criteria are met. On arrival, you will meet yet another set of nursing staff that might include a nurse and nursing assistants.

Have a discussion with your nurse regarding several items to make sure you are both on the same page:

- Establish a plan and a goal for pain levels. Again, zero is not a realistic plan. Be aware that some pain medications are ordered as needed, so you will have to ask for them.

- Establish a plan for sleep. One common complaint about the hospital stay is that you are often woken up during the night to take medications or to take your vital signs. Before you go to sleep, be sure to discuss the overnight plan for these things with your nurse. You might have the option for some "do not disturb" hours.

There are two common pieces of equipment used after a hip replacement for blood clot prevention. The first is compression stockings. These are usually white, tight-fitting hose that go from your foot to your thigh. Whether you use them is purely surgeon preference. I have stopped using them in my practice because of the lack of scientific data showing that they prevent blood clots or swelling. Some patients find them uncomfortable. If your surgeon prefers them, I would wear them. The second item commonly used is a pneumatic compression device or *sequential compression device (SCD)*. SCDs are sleeves that wrap around the calves or feet. An accompanying machine injects air periodically into the sleeves so that they squeeze your legs and/or feet. This improves blood flow in the veins and decreases the risk of DVT. I use these devices for my patients.

While you are in your hospital bed, I also recommend doing ankle pump exercises. Alternate pointing your toes toward the ceiling and the wall in front of you (Figure 10-1). Do sets of twenty or thirty at a time with both ankles several times throughout the day. This can also keep the blood moving in the legs.

Hospital policies differ on whether family or friends can stay overnight with you. If this is allowed, it is purely your choice. The hospital will have staff available to care for you.

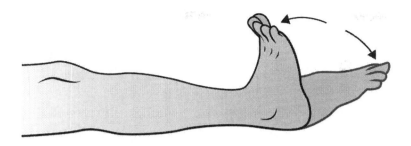

**Figure 10-1**: Ankle pumps – do these when resting.

---

**Fall Risk After Surgery**

Anyone who has had anesthesia and hip surgery is at risk for falls. A fall after hip replacement can be devastating, but it can be avoided with proper precautions. Never try to stand or walk without the assistance, especially in the first one to two days after surgery.

---

# Early Recovery Rules

There are some important rules to follow in early recovery. These start on the day of surgery and extend for several weeks after you are home:

1. **Ice**: It is hard to use too much ice, especially during the first two weeks. This can be bags of ice, an ice gel wrap, or an ice machine. If you use ice bags or a frozen gel wrap, make sure it's not in direct contact with the skin or it may burn the skin. If you've purchased an ice machine, ask if the hospital will allow you to use it during your stay. Don't focus on tracking the exact timing of ice on and off the hip, just keep it on most of the time when you are resting and take periodic breaks.

2. **Elevation**: Your thigh and lower leg will be swollen from surgery. This happens 100 percent of the time. There is no way to eliminate it. The best way to reduce swelling is with elevation. When you are in bed, on the couch, or sitting in a chair, a good rule of thumb is "toes above the nose." I recommend at least

three pillows under the knee and foot to get your toes to the proper height.

3.  **Weight-bearing restrictions:** Most of the time, patients are allowed to put full weight on their newly replaced hip. There are some scenarios where your surgeon will want to limit your weight-bearing to partial or no weight on the leg that had surgery. Make sure you and your therapist have clear instructions for this.

4.  **Hip dislocation precautions**: As mentioned in Chapter 6, the ball is at risk for popping out of the socket after surgery in every hip replacement patient. Luckily, it rarely happens, and careful precautions can decrease your risk. The early recovery period is the time when it's most susceptible to this. The further you are out from surgery, the lower the chance of a dislocation. You can avoid dislocation by paying attention to the position of your leg and foot. The type of precautions depends highly on your surgeon and the surgical approach. With any joint replacement surgery, NEVER STRETCH YOUR HIP in any direction during the first two to three months. Attempting to stretch your hip joint will not speed your recovery and may cause harm. Table 10-1 shows common anterior and posterior dislocation precautions:

**Table 10-1:** Positions to avoid after hip replacement surgery. Your surgeon or your therapist can tell you if these apply to you.

| Anterior Precautions (avoid) | Posterior Precautions (avoid) |
|---|---|
| Extending the operative leg backward | Crossing legs |
| Turning foot outward | Sitting in a low chair or toilet |
| | Bending at the waist past 90 degrees |
| | Bringing knee toward your chest |
| | Turning foot inward (try to keep it straight) |

## In-Hospital Therapy

The goals of the therapy team are to teach you how to get out of bed safely, the safest positions for your legs, introduce you to walking with a walker/crutch/cane, teach you how to dress and bathe, and to determine when you are ready to go home. I rely heavily on the therapy teams to tell me if patients require a rehab center stay after the hospital due to safety concerns.

Whereas therapy exercises are critical after knee replacement, I prefer minimal therapy exercises after hip replacement for the first six weeks. I see little advantage in doing repetitive strengthening exercises compared to simple walking, and some exercises have the potential for harm.

Stairs are a common concern for patients after surgery. However, patients rarely have problems once they learn the appropriate technique. The technique involves putting most of the load on your non-operative leg and taking stairs one at a time. Which leg is loaded depends on which direction you are heading. The therapists should coach you in this, but the rules are:

> Going up stairs:      lead with the non-operative leg
> Going down stairs:   lead with the operative leg

## Case Managers

A case manager or care coordinator may visit you during your hospital stay. The case manager is there to make sure that you have a safe place to go, have transportation home, have all the equipment you need, and provide resources for any other services outside the hospital. If you require a *skilled nursing facility* (or rehab center) after your hospital stay, your case manager may help you arrange that.

## Medical Team

Depending on your health history and hospital policies, you may have a team of medical providers visiting you in the hospital dedicated to watching over your health issues and medications outside the surgery site. Your surgeon is still in charge of surgical issues, but a medical team may assist the surgical team in managing conditions such as diabetes, heart conditions, and provide recommendations when any medical issues arise after surgery. I find their input invaluable, and always welcome their help.

## Criteria for Discharge to Home

Patients should have the same discharge criteria whether they go home on the day of surgery or they stay several nights. There are criteria that account for physical therapy goals, medical status, and making sure that the patient and the home situation is safe. Each hospital or surgery center has its own criteria, but Table 10-2 outlines some typical criteria used to make this decision.

## Education at Hospital Discharge

Once you meet your facility's discharge criteria, you will begin the discharge process. A critical component to discharge is education. Have a friend or family member present because there will be a lot of information to absorb. Make sure that you have a clear understanding of:

- **Your medications**: timing, dosages, which require prescriptions, which are over the counter, and when to start/stop each

- **Activity levels at home**: how much weight to put on your operative leg, range of motion restrictions, and recommended activity levels

- **Surgical dressing**: when/if you can shower, if it can get wet, and the plan for removal

- **Physical therapy**: what is the plan for your first appointment, will it be at home or at an outpatient center?

- **Surgeon follow-up**: know the date, time, and location

- **Contacts**: who and when to call with questions/concerns

**Table 10-2:** Typical Home Discharge Criteria

| Physical therapy criteria | • Walk thirty feet on level ground with a walker<br>• Walk up and down two to three stairs<br>• Demonstrate understanding of hip dislocation precautions<br>• Perform bathroom transfers<br>• Stand from a supine position in bed<br>• Be able to dress self and perform basic activities of daily living<br>• Equipment is available for home: walker, shower seat, etc. |
|---|---|
| Medical criteria | • Tolerate a solid food diet<br>• Pain reasonably controlled<br>• Vital signs stable<br>• No vomiting (mild nausea is common)<br>• Patient cleared for discharge by the surgical team<br>• Patient cleared for discharge by the medical team (if applicable)<br>• Able to urinate or catheter in place* |
| Patient criteria | • Confirm availability of full-time help at home for at least seventy-two hours<br>• Received education on medications and home care<br>• Patient has a driver/ride home<br>• Patient/family comfortable with discharge |

\* In rare cases, patients cannot urinate on their own and need to have a catheter placed, which will be removed after discharge.

## Pain Medications after Hip Replacement

The medications you take in the hospital will be similar to those you take at home. One advantage of staying overnight is that we have the opportunity to tinker with different pain medications to find the combination that works best for you.

Most surgeons endorse what we call *multimodal pain management*, which uses several medications that work on different pain pathways rather than big doses of single opioids. Medication types will differ between patients based on medical conditions.

Here are the most commonly prescribed options:

- **Opioids**: There is a major difference between pre- and post-surgery recommendations: opioid medications are appropriate for post-surgical pain. Commonly prescribed opioids include oxycodone (Percocet® or Oxycontin®), hydrocodone (Norco® or Vicodin®), morphine (MS Contin®), hydromorphone (Dilaudid®), and tramadol (Ultram®). Note that while opioids offer excellent pain control properties, they have more potential side effects than any other medication I prescribe.

- **NSAIDs**: Common options include prescription and non-prescription types including celecoxib (Celebrex®), meloxicam (Mobic®), ibuprofen (Advil® or Motrin), and naproxen (Aleve®)

- **Acetaminophen (Tylenol®):** This can be used as an adjunct medication to those above. Never take acetaminophen without discussing it with your medical team because some other medications may already have acetaminophen in them.

---

### Common Side Effects of Opioids

Side effects are so significant in some patients that they are worse than the pain from surgery. If side effects cannot be counteracted, you may have to choose between pain and taking these medications.

- Nausea: if you have consistent nausea after surgery, this is the most likely culprit
- Constipation: everyone taking them should be on laxatives and stool softeners
- Dizziness, somnolence, mental cloudiness
- Skin itching or hives
- Dry mouth
- Moodiness
- Hallucinations
- Difficulty with urination
- Respiratory depression (slowed, shallow breathing) – overdose can cause death

## Other Common Medications
## after Hip Replacement

Most of the other medications given after hip replacement are to counteract the side effects of the surgery or the other medications. Commonly suggested medications include:

- **Blood-thinning agent**: This is surgeon and patient-dependent, and can be aspirin, a medication injected under the skin, or one of many other pill formulations. This usually starts on the day of surgery or the day after surgery. How long to take this medication varies by the surgeon and the patient, and ranges from two to six weeks after surgery.

- **Laxatives and Stool Softeners:** If you are on opioid pain medications, you are at high risk for constipation or a more serious problem such as bowel obstruction. There are several formulations that can be purchased over the counter, and you may need to take more than one. Ask your medical team or pharmacist what is best for you.

- **Stomach acid blockers:** If you are on an NSAID or higher doses of aspirin, stomach acid blockers may be recommended to avoid stomach irritation or even stomach ulcers. There are both over the counter and prescription options. Discuss with your medical providers first.

- **Anti-nausea medications**: Nausea is common after anesthesia and with opioid pain medications. There are some IV and oral options to counteract nausea.

## Where to Go After Hospital Discharge

There are generally two options for where to go after hospital discharge. The first is a rehab center, which is also called a *skilled nursing facility* or *SNF*. This is a care center where you go and stay with twenty-four-hour care available. Meals are prepared for you and you undergo daily physical therapy. The second option is your own home.

I strongly advise you to make every effort to go home. Historically, more patients have gone to a rehab center, but the current trend is moving away from this option. While the idea of twenty-four-hour care might sound like a good idea, there are several clear downsides. First, studies show that patients who go to a rehab center have more complications and more hospital readmissions. Just like the hospital, the rehab center exposes you to infection, and you submit to others caring for you, which leads to passive recovery. Remember we want active recovery, not passive.

A small subset of patients with significantly impaired mobility or medical problems need closer attention than the home environment provides. If it is truly not safe to go home but you don't need the level of medical care that a hospital provides, then a rehab center is a good choice.

## Chapter 10 Review

- Plan for a short stay in the hospital – there are many advantages to going home.

- Develop a plan for pain medications and sleep with your nurses in the hospital.

- Never attempt to stand or walk on your own. Falling is a significant risk after surgery.

- Ice, elevation, and walking are all important in early recovery.

- Physical therapists, occupational therapists, a case manager, and medical hospitalists may be involved in your care.

- Specific discharge criteria must be met whether you are having surgery at a surgery center or a hospital.

- Make sure you have a clear understanding of your discharge instructions and who to call before leaving the hospital.

- Where you go after surgery depends on your medical conditions and your overall function. Aim to go home rather than a rehab center if this is safe for you.

Chapter Eleven

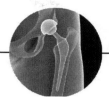

# Recovery
## *The First 12 Weeks after Surgery*

Your surgery is done, and you've got a new hip. I tell my patients that the surgery and the time in the hospital or surgery center are the easy part because you are guided through every step and the work is done for you. It is now your turn to put in some effort and start taking charge of your own care and your own outcome. Let us go through what to expect at each time point along the way.

## Your Own Journey

This was mentioned at the beginning of Chapter 1, and it's worth repeating. You will recover from hip replacement differently than anyone else. In fact, if you have both of your hips replaced at different points in time, those will be two different experiences. I strongly urge you to not compare yourself to others. You will recover more quickly/easily than some and will experience more difficulty than others. If you are concerned about progress, ask your surgeon or your therapist. They will not be bashful about telling you if you are not on track.

## Passive Versus Active Recovery

*Passive recovery* consists of lying in bed or on the couch all day, having others wait on you, and moving little. We have learned that getting up on your feet and moving around after surgery decreases complications and speeds the recovery process. *Active recovery* includes getting up and walking around several times per day and increasing your activity with time.

Let's be clear on one point: you can overdo it. If you overdo it, you will have a setback in the recovery process. Your body needs time to heal, so listen to it. How much to move around and how far to walk varies from patient to patient. Start with being on your feet three to five times per day indoors for a few minutes with someone assisting you to avoid falls and increase SLOWLY from there.

## Pain Management at Home

Most patients need opioids for a short period of time after hip replacement. Opioids are good for short-term post-surgical pain control if patients can handle the many side effects.

It is well published that we have an opioid epidemic in the United States. We consume eighty percent of the world's prescription opioids despite having less than five percent of the world population. We use far more opioids before and after surgery than other countries. Overdoses and visits to the emergency department are too common. The data is clear: we are overusing and abusing these drugs. Patients and doctors both play a role in this. Orthopedic surgeons prescribe eight percent of the narcotic pain medications, which puts us fourth on the list of all prescribers. I am constantly examining my opioid prescribing methods and encourage other medical providers to do the same.

Opioids are terrible long-term pain relievers. Some studies estimate the addiction risk after short-term use is up to forty-five percent, and if taken for more than twelve weeks, there is a fifty percent chance a patient will be using them at five years. They can change your life and your personality for the worse.

The bottom line is this: **get off opioids as soon as possible.** Transition to NSAIDs or acetaminophen as early as you can tolerate the transition. Timing is different for every patient. I have some patients who never use them after hip replacement. MOST patients can come off them after one or two weeks. I now use great scrutiny in providing them beyond four weeks and will rarely prescribe them after six weeks.

# Leg Bruising and Swelling

Most patients bruise after hip replacement. Some bruise a lot. Bruising forms around the thigh and the hip, and with time, follows gravity toward the foot. The bruising usually starts out black, blue, or purple, and with time colors change to a lighter blue, yellow, maybe even orangish or greenish. There is nothing you can do to avoid or remove bruising other than to give it time. This is an important expectation to set: there is no amount of bruising that is concerning after hip replacement. Bruising alone never indicates a problem.

All patients have swelling after hip replacement. The location of swelling is similar to bruising – it can be anywhere from the thigh to the toes. Swelling can be a source of pain. When the skin and other soft tissues stretch from swelling, it causes a painful sensation. Swelling is something you can reduce with ice and elevation. Elevation of the feet (remember, "toes above the nose") is the best way to decrease swelling.

A caveat to swelling needs to be discussed briefly. Swelling and calf pain can be signs of a blood clot in the legs (DVT). This is difficult to diagnose and interpret because we just established that everyone has swelling in the legs. New-onset pain in the calf is one sign to watch out for. It is difficult to give advice on when to seek help for this, and every surgeon has a slightly different protocol. My best advice is to discuss the protocol for diagnosing DVT with your surgeon to find out when he or she would want to be notified.

# Incision, Surgical Dressing, and Bathing

Surgeons often have strict preferences on how the surgical dressing and incision are handled. Follow your surgeon's instructions closely. Some close the incision with staples and some with *sutures* (stitches). Staples need to be removed and sutures are often absorbable and do not require removal. Some surgeons use skin glue in addition to sutures to seal and reinforce the incision. The skin glue is like Super Glue® but made for medical applications.

Some surgical dressings are water-resistant, while others are not. Those that are water-resistant may allow for showering but not baths, hot tubs, or swimming pools. **Check with your surgeon when showering and bathing are allowed.** To be safe you can use a combination of clear plastic kitchen wrap and medical tape to wrap in the shower (not bath) and protect it from the water.

The timing to remove the surgical dressing is also highly surgeon-dependent. Some surgeons will change the surgical dressing in the hospital, and others will not. Some may have you remove it at home. Some may want to remove it in their office. Please follow their guidelines closely.

Do not let the appearance of your incision worry you in the first few weeks. The hip can be red, swollen, painful, and might even look "angry". Surgeons spend a lot of time educating patients and even other medical providers about what a normal postoperative incision looks like because it may frighten those who don't see them regularly. Be assured that the only definitive sign of early infection is persistent wound drainage, and it is rarely diagnosed in the first week after surgery. Contact your surgeon if you have any concerns.

Do not put any lotions, oils, rubs, ointments, or any other home remedy on your incision without clearance from your surgeon. Patients often want to get vitamin E or another scar-minimizing ointment on the scar as early as possible. There is no good evidence to suggest that these formulations do anything to decrease scar appearance in early recovery, so listen to your surgeon's recommendations.

## Therapy Outside the Hospital

Whereas formal physical therapy immediately following surgery is a requirement for my patients after knee replacement, I prefer no therapy for the first six weeks after hip replacement. My philosophy is to let the soft tissues heal and allow the new hip joint to solidify, then work on strengthening after things have settled down. Some surgeons feel strongly about initiating therapy immediately after surgery, and you should follow their recommendations.

After six weeks, you may benefit from strengthening exercises and gait training. If you had a limp before surgery, you need to retrain your muscles to walk without a limp after surgery. This takes weeks to months in some cases. Physical therapists can give you tips on how to avoid limping and exercises to strengthen chronically weak muscles.

## Urgent Conditions

One reason to be checked out immediately is persistent blood or other fluid drainage from the incision, which may fill up the dressing. Other urgent issues are medical conditions that should concern you with or without surgery. If you have chest pain, breathing problems, or you pass out, call 911. You should be seen immediately if you have uncontrollable vomiting or diarrhea, persistent fever over $101^0$ F, significant abdominal pain, or new/unrelenting calf pain or swelling. Your surgeon or the hospital should give you a list of reasons to call, and that list should supersede this list.

## What to Expect During Weeks 0-2

The first two weeks after hip replacement are often the most difficult. The level of difficulty varies from patient to patient, but this is the hardest time for most everyone. The good news is that if you expect and prepare for it, you will get through it just fine, and it will get better! Every day will be a step toward a better hip and life. Focus on ice, elevation, brief standing/walking, rest, stay positive, and then repeat.

| | |
|---|---|
| **Swelling**: | Typically increases around the incision over the first one to two weeks. Follow foot elevation and icing protocols (toes above nose!) |
| **Pain Control**: | Most patients will need some opioid pain medication and other adjunct medications. Use opioids for the shortest time possible and try to discontinue them in one to two weeks if you can. |
| **Activity**: | Early on, aim to get up and walk three to five times per day. You can start to do this at home initially. Later, when you can do so comfortably and safely, you can take some short walks outside. Do not overdo it – you might have a setback that delays your recovery. |

| **DVT prevention**: | Your primary blood clot prevention is movement, walking, and ankle pump exercises. Most patients should also be on some form of medication to prevent blood clots during the first two weeks or more after surgery. |
| **Appointments**: | Most surgeons will want to see you within the first two weeks after surgery. They may have an assistant in their office see you on their behalf. The purpose of your first appointment is to check your incision, educate you, answer questions, and reassure you. |

## What to Expect During Weeks 2-6

You should start to see progress. Pain should be decreasing, and you should gradually return to your normal routine.

| **Swelling:** | Should be decreasing but you may still have swelling around the hip, and possibly in the foot and ankle at six weeks after surgery. |
| **Pain Control:** | Decrease or remove opioid pain medications from your pain control regimen. Few patients should still be on them four to six weeks post-surgery. If you are still on them at six weeks, discuss other options with your medical providers. |
| **Activity:** | Start to resume some of your daily routine. Patients often return to work and might be driving themselves in the two-to-six week range. See the discussion later in this chapter on work and driving. Walking distance varies by patient, but most should be increasing outdoor walking distance. Do not overdo it – you might have a setback that delays your recovery. |
| **DVT prevention**: | Your primary blood clot risk drops after two weeks, but you should still be using activity to prevent them. Depending on your surgeon's medication protocols, you may still be on a blood thinner during this time. |
| **Appointments**: | Most surgeons will want to see you between four and six weeks. |

# What to Expect During Weeks 6-12

By weeks six to twelve, you should really like your new hip. But will it be fully recovered? Not yet. We will discuss in the final chapter what full recovery looks like and how long it takes.

Most patients are quite satisfied with the hip by the time they are three months out, and the good news is that it just keeps getting better after that. On average, patients are 80-90 percent recovered at twelve weeks, which means most of the recovery occurs in the first three months; however, there is still room for improvement.

| | |
|---|---|
| **Swelling:** | Should be decreasing and minimal in most patients by twelve weeks post-op. |
| **Pain Control:** | You should be off opiates, and off most of the other pain medications as well. Some patients use occasional over-the-counter pain relievers at this point. Instead of taking scheduled doses, most patients can begin to take medications as needed. |
| **Activity:** | You should be back to your daily routine, most are back to work, most are driving, and walking longer distances outdoors should not be limited by your hip. |
| **Range of motion:** | Continue to be careful with stretching your hip. It's not fully healed yet. You may notice that putting on your socks and shoes is becoming easier, and that continues to improve naturally with time. |
| **Physical therapy:** | If you believe you have strength deficits or gait abnormalities and have not yet started with a therapist, now is a good time to discuss it with your surgeon. |
| **DVT prevention:** | At this point, your risk of a blood clot is close to what it was before surgery, so most patients can discontinue blood-thinning medications unless your medical providers advise otherwise, or you have underlying conditions that require them. |
| **Appointments:** | Some surgeons want to see their patients at about three months out from surgery, though this is not universal. |

## Driving

Time to return to driving varies by patient. There are two criteria that you must meet before driving after hip surgery. First, you must be off all medications that might impede your ability to drive. This is primarily the opioid pain medications. Second, you must be able to operate the vehicle safely. This second criterion is completely up to you since your medical providers won't be able to observe you in a driving situation.

For vehicles with automatic transmission, your right foot is typically your gas-brake foot. This means that if you've had left hip surgery and are off pain medications, you may be able to drive safely right away. For right hip surgery or a vehicle with a manual transmission, it might take weeks to drive safely. Studies have shown that around four weeks after surgery most patients can push the brake pedal with normal reaction times. Make sure you can safely do this before you get behind the wheel. Get the blessing of your loved ones and test your driving safety in a vacant parking lot before you resume driving.

## Returning to Work

Returning to work is another individualized goal that varies greatly from patient to patient. Patients who own businesses or have no alternative income while they are out for surgery tend to go back earlier than those that have sick time or temporary disability policies in place. Heavy laborers need more time off work than those with desk jobs. Preoperative function and postoperative pain levels also predict your return to work. Some patients start working immediately after surgery if they can work remotely and can sit for work. Some work a part-time schedule on initial return, while others wait until they can return full-time. This is your decision that you should discuss with your surgeon, your family, and your employer.

From a symptomatic standpoint, there are three things that might limit you from returning to work. The first is obvious – hip pain. The more you are on your feet doing other things, the more it is likely to swell and hurt, especially early in recovery. Secondly, hip replacement drains your energy for a few weeks. Patients report having more fatigue in early recovery than they had before surgery. Third, some jobs might not be safe to return because of physical limitations (think first-responders, laborers, need to climb ladders, etc.).

The following are averages of when patients generally return to work after hip replacement:

- Sedentary job with limited hours or remote work option: zero to four weeks

- Sedentary job, at an office location, full-time: three to eight weeks

- Non-laborer, but the job requires substantial walking/standing: four to eight weeks

- Laborer, first-responder, or need to climb ladders: eight to twelve weeks

## Travel after Hip Replacement

Historically, orthopedic surgeons have limited travel in the initial weeks after hip replacement due to concerns for blood clots with prolonged sitting in a confined space. However, recent studies show that there is no significant increased risk of blood clots with post-surgery travel. Some surgeons have held onto strict travel restrictions. You should check and see what your surgeon's recommendations are on this subject.

If you do travel, the best advice is to get up and move around frequently. Other common recommendations include the use of compression stockings, stretching your leg muscles, doing calf squeezes and ankle pumps, and staying well hydrated.

## Chapter 11 Review

- Hip replacement is your own journey. Resist the temptation to compare yourself to others.

- Get off opioid pain medications as soon as you are able.

- Bruising and swelling are extremely common after hip replacement and can occur anywhere from the thigh to the foot.

- Follow your surgeon's surgical dressing, showering, and bathing recommendations closely.

- The first two weeks after surgery are the hardest, but things improve after that.

- At four to six weeks out from surgery, most people are back to their normal routine and off opioid pain medications

- By twelve weeks, your hip feels substantially better, but you are not 100 percent healed or improved or recovered yet.

- Full recovery can take six to twelve months after hip replacement.

Chapter Twelve

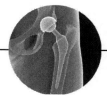

# Beyond 12 Weeks

## *Achieving Full Recovery*

After twelve weeks, your hip will continue to improve. Pain should decrease with time. If you had a limp before surgery, it should slowly resolve. The ultimate goal is to be able to work, exercise, and rest without noticing your hip. Your new hip will be at its best when you achieve full recovery.

## What is "Full Recovery"?

Full recovery is a state of maximum improvement. This state varies for every patient. Some patients will have minimal pain complaints and/or symptoms. Patients consistently say they are satisfied and that their hips are significantly better than before surgery, but not every hip is pain-free and symptom-free. If you've done your part, your strength and function will recover over time.

Leading into surgery, if you had significant weakness, difficulty walking, a substantial limp, or limiting medical conditions, these factors prolong your recovery. The hip replacement reconstructs your joint surfaces but not the muscles and other soft tissues that surround the hip joint.

In most patients, a state of maximum improvement occurs between six and twelve months post-surgery. I've seen it take eighteen months in some patients. Time is important in reaching this state, but you can speed it along by keeping the hip strong and staying active.

## Continuing Physical Therapy

Some patients have significant strength deficits or gait abnormalities from years of hip arthritis. Other patients are able to strengthen and rehab their hip by resuming their daily routine. If you have questions about your hip function or strength, it might be worth a consultation and evaluation with a physical therapist.

## Antibiotics for Dental Visits and Other Procedures

There is much debate in the orthopedic and dental communities as to whether joint replacement patients should take antibiotics before dental procedures. I have read through the available literature, talked to dentists and other surgeons, and the only thing that's clear is that there is no consensus. There are strong feelings on both sides of the subject. Everyone seems to agree that dental procedures release some normal mouth bacteria into the bloodstream. What is not clear is whether these bacteria cause artificial joint infections. The American Dental Association lists the following statement on their website:

> In patients with prosthetic joint implants, a January 2015 ADA clinical practice guideline, based on a 2014 systematic review states, "In general, for patients with prosthetic joint implants, prophylactic antibiotics are not recommended prior to dental procedures to prevent prosthetic joint infection"[10].

I must agree with the dentists here; the scientific studies generally show that the risk of infection of artificial joints is extremely low. Taking antibiotics may be unnecessary.

The other side of the argument is generally led by orthopedic surgeons. Most surgeons who do high-volume joint replacements have seen patients show up with joint infections shortly after a dental procedure. When this happens, the dentist usually does not hear about it and the situation can be threatening to the patient's limb. Some orthopedic surgeons' position is that a single dose of antibiotics is low risk and might prevent a disastrous infection.

My suggestion is that you talk with your surgeon and come up with a plan that you are both comfortable with.

# When to See Your Surgeon

Most surgeons want patients to check in with them yearly, especially if they have enrolled you in research studies. I have found that yearly evaluation for happy patients is not necessary. If you are happy with your hip replacement, the chance of finding something abnormal that we are going to correct is low. I think it's reasonable for happy patients to space out appointments every three to five years, but you should discuss recommendations with your surgeon. You should book an appointment with your surgeon if you notice a change in pain or other symptoms that don't resolve over time.

There are no reliable signs of infection after hip replacement except for fluid drainage that occurs after the incision is initially healed. Fluid coming out of a previously healed incision or near a joint replacement incision is infection until proven otherwise. Contact your surgeon if you see this.

# Longevity

One of the most common questions surgeons are asked is how long hip replacements last. This is a bit of a guess because we are using the best materials we have ever used, and there are many manufacturers, materials, and techniques. Based on available studies, we can expect most modern hip replacements to last twenty to thirty years. A low percentage will fail before twenty years and failures are unpredictable in both cause and timing. Reasons for failure could be plastic wear, loosening of metal parts, infection, instability, or stiffness. Chances are that yours will last you many years, and for most patients, one hip replacement is all they will ever need.

## Chapter 12 Review

- The time to full recovery varies from patient to patient, but most reach maximum improvement at six to twelve months after surgery.

- Occasional aches, pains, and swelling can be normal symptoms, especially in the first year after hip replacement.

- If you want the best possible hip function, develop a program that involves both strength and cardiovascular components to get the most out of your hip and to maximize your overall health.

- Whether to take antibiotics before dental visits is a decision you should discuss with your surgeon.

- Most hip replacements last twenty to thirty years.

# Appendix

## Hip Strengthening Exercises

**CAUTION**: Wait until your surgeon and therapist clear you to do exercises after surgery. I prefer that my patients do nothing but simple walking for at least six weeks after hip replacement. In some cases, trying to do exercises too early can cause problems and setbacks.

The following exercises can be safely done BEFORE surgery. In most cases, these are safe to start twelve weeks after surgery, but again, check with your surgeon to make sure they are safe for you.

**Squats:** These strengthen the quadriceps, gluteal muscles, and the hamstrings. Do whichever variant is most comfortable for you.

1. <u>Standing squat</u>: With both arms extended outward for balance, try to keep your back upright and bend at the knees. It is important not to bend over at the waist. If you have to bend at the waist do not do squats. Go down only as far as you can comfortably, but never past a 90-degree bend in the knees or the hips.

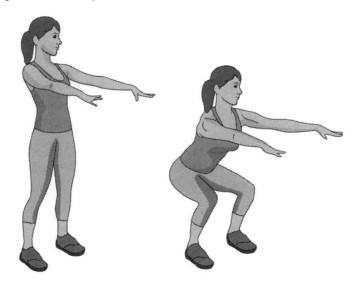

2. <u>Chair assisted squat</u>: Some people find using a chair as a reference point helpful. Higher chairs or a bed can decrease how far you need to bend your knees. Limit bending forward at the waist. Try to keep your back straight up and down. If you need to bend at the waist then assist with your hands on your thighs or skip chair squats altogether.

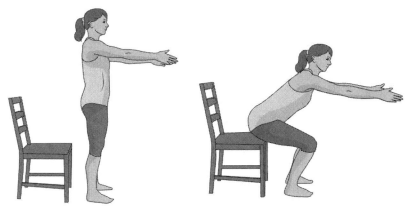

3. <u>Wall sits</u>: Using a wall for stabilization is easier for some patients than squatting up and down. Do not do these if you are concerned about getting back to a standing position. Set goal times and increase as you get stronger.

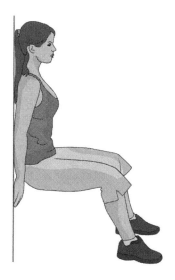

**Standing Hamstring Curls:** Using a chair or rail for balance, lift one foot off the ground so the knee is bent 90 degrees, hold a few seconds at the top, and return the foot to the floor. You can add ankle weights to increase resistance. Do three sets of fifteen curls for each leg at least three days per week.

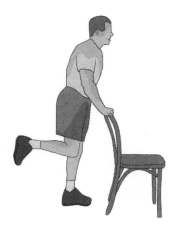

**Lateral Leg Lifts:** Lateral leg lifts can promote strength in some key muscles around the hip joint. Lying on your side, hold your leg straight and lift to an angle of 45 degrees with the ground, hold for two seconds, then lower your straight leg to the floor slowly. Aim for three sets of fifteen for each leg at least three days per week.

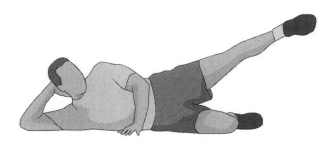

**Clamshells:** Lie on your side with hips flexed slightly forward and knees bent. Raise the top knee off the bottom knee while keeping your feet together. Lower slowly back down. Repeat 10-15 times.

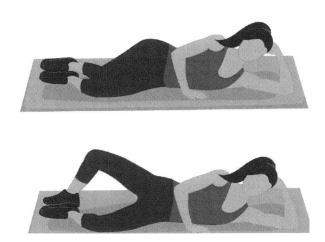

# Frequently Asked Questions

**Should I ask my surgeon if he or she uses recalled products?** I can say with confidence that nobody uses recalled instruments or joint replacement parts. It would be a setup for a lawsuit to knowingly use recalled products, and in the United States use of anything recalled or defective is monitored by hospitals, government agencies, companies selling the products, and the surgeons themselves. This should not be an issue.

**Do I need a special card or note for airport security after hip replacement?** There are no special cards or notes for airport security after hip surgery. Let TSA agents know that you have an artificial joint, and they will direct you to appropriate screening processes.

**Can someone take videos or photos of my surgery?** Most hospitals have policies that don't allow photos or videos in the operating room.

**Can I keep any of my own bone, cartilage, or ligaments removed from the hip at the time of surgery?** Most hospitals have strict policies against this, and they are typically disposed of in a sterile manner.

**What is the recovery time after hip replacement?** Remember, everyone is different. I tell patients it takes, on average, four to six weeks to return to most normal activities. Assume you will be 80 to 90 percent recovered three months after surgery. Most people require six to twelve months to reach a point of maximum improvement with respect to swelling, pain, and function.

**What about sex after hip replacement?** This is a common question. American Academy of Hip and Knee Surgeons put together an excellent guide with illustrations of safe positions. Please check out their website: https://hipknee.aahks.org/a-guide-to-returning-to-sexual-activity-following-total-hip-and-knee-replacement/

**Can I go up and down stairs after total hip replacement surgery?** There are typically no restrictions to stairs after hip replacement and most patients can navigate stairs within a day or two after the procedure. Discuss the technique for going up and down stairs with your therapist.

**Do I need antibiotics before dental work after my hip is replaced?** This a controversial topic and depends on your history, your surgeon, and your dentist. See Chapter 12 for more information.

**Do I need special antibiotics for other invasive procedures after total hip replacement surgery?** In general, you don't need anything special, but it's always best to check with your surgeon for specific circumstances.

**Do I need antibiotics when I get a cold or flu after total hip replacement surgery?** Your hip replacement should not change your need for antibiotics with common illnesses. Your primary care provider should guide your use of antibiotics for cold or flu symptoms.

**Is a feeling of depression normal after hip replacement?** Yes! I believe this is underappreciated by patients and the medical community. The stress of surgery and the medications we typically give can make you feel tired and depressed for a period of weeks. Coming off the opiate pain medications can also cause symptoms of depression.

**Is insomnia normal after hip replacement?** Yes! Despite feeling tired, many patients have difficulty sleeping because of pain or medication side effects. Mindfulness exercises and a discussion with your primary care provider can help if insomnia does not improve with time.

**How long will my total hip replacement last?** Recent studies show that more than 80 percent of hip replacements will survive more than twenty years.

**Can I get an MRI after hip replacement?** Yes. The metal parts in the hip will not have any effect on the MRI in most cases. Just let the radiology team know that you have a hip replacement.

**I had hip replacement three months ago and it still hurts while my friend's hip did not hurt at three months. Is this normal?** There are two important points that I hope this book drills home because understanding them will affect your recovery and satisfaction. First, it takes six to twelve months for maximum improvement of symptoms, so most patients will still have pain or discomfort at three months. Second, everyone recovers at a different rate, so resist the temptation to compare your recovery to others.

# Preoperative Checklist

- ❑ Identify your joint coach, help for home, and a driver after surgery.
- ❑ Schedule the surgery date.
- ❑ Verify with your insurance company that the surgery is covered.
- ❑ Develop a plan for mental preparation (meditation, various cognitive therapies, see a mental health provider if needed).
- ❑ Develop a plan for physical preparation (hip exercises and/or aerobic exercises).
- ❑ Develop a healthy diet plan before surgery.
- ❑ Develop a food plan for after surgery (frozen meals or have someone to cook for you).
- ❑ Search for and remove hazards for tripping, slipping, or falling in the home (rugs, cords, toys, and even small animals).
- ❑ Purchase or borrow a walker and a cane.
- ❑ Consider purchasing or borrowing an ice machine.
- ❑ Have a plan for icing at home: ice machine, gel packs, frozen vegetables, or plastic bags with ice in them.
- ❑ Schedule your preoperative history and physical (must be within thirty days of surgery). Check with your surgeon to see if you should use a special clinic or your primary care provider.
- ❑ Complete labs and other ordered studies well before the surgery date.
- ❑ If you smoke, stop at least six weeks prior to surgery. Use this as your reason to quit forever.
- ❑ If you are diabetic, keep blood sugars under good control leading up to surgery.

❏ Limit alcohol use to two drinks or less per day in the weeks leading up to surgery. Do not drink any alcohol for two days before your procedure.

❏ If you use opiate pain medications, stop them at least four weeks prior to surgery. Have the prescribing medical provider help you taper off them well before surgery.

❏ Schedule a joint replacement class (if one is available).

❏ Your surgeon, your primary care provider, or the clinic you go to for your preoperative medical appointment should give you a list of medications to stop before surgery. Pay attention to this list as it's important.

❏ If your body mass index is more than thirty and you have time before surgery, work on weight loss. Do not go on a "crash diet" just prior to surgery.

❏ If you have not seen a dentist in the six months leading up to surgery, it's a good idea to get a checkup and cleaning. Don't have any dental work done in the two weeks prior to surgery.

❏ Make sure your vaccines are up to date well before surgery (flu, pneumonia, etc.). New flu vaccines are available in the early fall each year. Don't get any vaccinations within two weeks of your surgery date.

❏ Schedule your first postoperative appointment with your surgeon's office.

❏ Look at the list of "Items to Bring with You" in Chapter 9.

❏ Write your current medications (including dosages), supplements, and medication allergies on a piece of paper to bring with you to surgery.

❏ Put clean sheets on your bed in preparation for your arrival home.

# Other Resources

## <u>Hip Arthritis</u>
### American Academy of Orthopaedic Surgeons (AAOS)
- The largest orthopedic organization in the world has an excellent patient education website that has hundreds of articles, videos, and other resources for bone and joint health: https://www.orthoinfo.org/

### American Association of Hip and Knee Surgeons (AAHKS)
- You can find a lot of valuable patient information on arthritis as well as hip and knee replacements: hipknee.aahks.org

- AAHKS as some position statements on topics such as stem cell therapies and opioid use here: www.aahks.org/position-statements

### American College of Rheumatology (ACR)
- A high-quality resource on various types of arthritis, particularly inflammatory conditions such as rheumatoid arthritis:

  www.rheumatology.org/I-Am-A/Patient-Caregiver

## <u>Mental Health and Meditation Books</u>

*10% Happier* by Dan Harris, 2014.
If you are unfamiliar with meditation and mindfulness, this is an easy read and a great place to start.

*The Power of Now* by Eckhart Tolle, 1999.
Tolle is a visionary, teacher, and influential leader in the world of mindfulness. This book starts strong and then repeats some themes, but it has the potential to be life-changing.

*Cognitive Behavioral Therapy Made Simple* by Seth J. Gillihan, Ph.D., 2018.
There is some evidence that this type of therapy can help with post-operative pain. This book requires more effort than those listed above. It has strategies and exercises that may strengthen mental wellness and prepare you for surgery.

# Hip Replacement Glossary

| | |
|---|---|
| **AAHKS** | American Association of Hip and Knee Surgeons |
| **AAOS** | American Academy of Orthopaedic Surgeons |
| **acetabulum** | The hip socket which is in the bony pelvis. |
| **active recovery** | Recovery from surgery that involves taking charge of your own care and moving around periodically. Contrast this with passive recovery. |
| **albumin** | A lab test that measures protein in the blood and serves as a surrogate for overall nutritional status. |
| **anecdotal evidence** | A very low level of scientific evidence that supports the use of a particular treatment based on experience but in the absence of true scientific study or peer-reviewed publications. |
| **arthritis** | An inflamed joint, usually with pain. |
| **arthron** | A Greek word meaning "joint". |
| **arthroplasty** | A term that describes reshaping a joint, or what we commonly call joint replacement. |
| **articular cartilage** | Surface cartilage in the hip joint. This covers the femoral head and acetabular surfaces. It provides a very smooth and slick surface to facilitate joint motion with low friction. |
| **articulate** | To form a joint. To rub together. |
| **autoimmune** | A disease whereby the body produces an inflammatory reaction against normal cells. |
| **ball and socket joint** | A joint where a ball rotates inside of a socket to give a large degree of motion. The hip and shoulder joints are ball and socket joints. |
| **bearing surfaces** | The two surfaces in a hip replacement that rub together (the femoral head and the liner in the acetabular cup). |
| **body mass index** | A formula used to assess obesity that takes into account a patient's height and weight. |

| | |
|---|---|
| **bone cyst** | A cavity that forms in the underlying bone as cartilage wears away in the hip joint. |
| **bone on bone arthritis** | An x-ray finding where all the cartilage space is gone on x-ray, and bones normally separated by cartilage are touching each other. |
| **bony pelvis** | The sacrum and two innominate bones found in the lower part of the trunk between the abdomen and the legs. The pelvis contains the hip socket (acetabulum). |
| **bronchitis** | Inflamed bronchi (tubes in the lungs). |
| **cartilage** | A substance found in joints that serves to protect the ends of two bones forming a joint. |
| **cartilage space narrowing** | Loss of cartilage space in the hip joint, seen on x-ray or other imaging studies. |
| **chronic** | A persistent or long-term condition (versus "acute" which describes a short-term condition). |
| **colitis** | An inflamed colon. |
| **components** | The metal and plastic parts that we put in the hip for hip replacement surgery. |
| **corticosteroid** | See steroid. This is a synonym for steroid and cortisone. |
| **cortisone** | See steroid. This is a synonym for steroid and corticosteroid. |
| **deep vein thrombosis** | A blood clot that occurs in the limbs during or after surgery. |
| **dislocation** | The femoral ball unexpectedly pops out of the socket after a hip replacement surgery. |
| **DVT** | Abbreviation for deep vein thrombosis. |
| **expert opinion** | An article published in a medical journal that often lacks significant scientific evidence but represents the opinion of an expert in the field of study. |

| | |
|---|---|
| **fellowship** | A one-year, specialized training program that surgeons may opt to complete after residency training. |
| **femoral canal** | The hollow interior of the femur shaft that is filled with bone marrow. We remove the marrow and place the prosthetic femoral stem in the canal. |
| **femoral head** | The top of the femur—the round ball that makes up the ball part of the ball and socket joint of the hip. |
| **femoral neck** | The segment of bone that connects the femoral head to the rest of the femur. |
| **femoral stem** | The metal piece of a hip replacement that is inserted into the canal of the femur. |
| **femur** | The thigh bone. The longest bone in the body. |
| **flare** | A short-term but intense increase in arthritis pain and inflammation. |
| **groin** | An area between the top of the thigh and lower abdomen where pain is commonly found when the hip joint is the cause. Also known as the inguinal crease. |
| **hemoglobin** | The substance in red blood cells that carries oxygen. The amount of hemoglobin is measurable with a lab test. |
| **hemoglobin A1c** | A blood test used to assess sugar levels in the blood, primarily in diabetic patients. |
| **inflammation** | The body's local response to injury or wear that is typically associated with swelling, pain, and warmth. |
| **inflammatory arthritis** | A form of arthritis where the body causes abnormal inflammation in a joint, typically due to an underlying autoimmune disorder such as rheumatoid arthritis. |
| **inguinal crease** | The crease between the top of the thigh and the lower abdomen. Also known as the groin. |

| | |
|---|---|
| **inherent** | Things you are born with or cannot change. |
| **-itis** | A suffix used in medicine that means "inflammation". |
| **labrum** | A fibrocartilage ring around the acetabulum (hip socket) that serves to cushion and seal the joint. |
| **lateral** | Away from the midline of the body. |
| **ligaments** | Strong, fibrous, soft tissue structures that connect two bones together. |
| **medial** | Toward the midline of the body. |
| **medical clearance** | A less desirable term for the medical optimization process that occurs around the time of surgery. |
| **medications** | Chemical compounds that are regulated by the FDA and used for the purpose of treating diseases or symptoms. |
| **metal-on-metal** | A metal femoral head (ball) that is used with a metal acetabular liner (socket). This construct is rarely used because of problems with shedding of metal ions. |
| **mild arthritis** | Mild inflammation or minimal cartilage space narrowing in a joint, usually, but not always, associated with mild symptoms. |
| **mindfulness** | A state of living whereby we guide ourselves to live in the moment. |
| **minimally invasive** | A surgical approach is called minimally invasive if it makes a smaller than standard skin incision and avoids splitting individual muscles. The exact definition is debated. |
| **moderate arthritis** | A condition in between mild and severe arthritis. Typically, at least half of the cartilage space is gone on x-ray. |
| **modifiable** | Things you can change. |
| **multifactorial** | Many factors contribute to a condition. |

**multimodal pain management**

Several medications that work by different mechanisms are used to control pain rather than large doses of a single medication.

**muscles**

Muscles around the hip joint not only help you stand and walk, but they help hold the hip joint together.

**NSAIDs**

Non-steroidal anti-inflammatory drugs (examples are ibuprofen and naproxen).

**occupational therapist**

A therapist who has expertise in performing activities of daily living and self-care after surgery.

**opioid-induced hyperalgesia**

A phenomenon that occurs when patients are exposed to opioid pain medications and pain receptors become more sensitive to pain over time.

**osteoarthritis**

The most common form of arthritis, typically described as "wear and tear" arthritis.

**osteophytes**

Bone spurs that can be found around the hip ball and socket when arthritis is present.

**osteoporosis**

Decreased density of the bones which occurs naturally with age, more prominent in females than males.

**pain**

An optional feature of arthritis. Not every joint with arthritis has pain.

**passive recovery**

Recovery from surgery that involves lying around all day and having others wait on your every need.

**patient testimonies**

Individual patients provide testimony that a particular treatment was effective for them.

**PE**

Abbreviation for pulmonary embolism.

**peer-reviewed**

A scientific study that has been reviewed by a professional peer with expertise in the subject matter of that study. This is done before publication in medical journals.

| | |
|---|---|
| **placebo effect** | A commonly accepted effect that occurs when only the idea of a treatment has the proposed effect of the treatment. |
| **-plasty** | A Greek word meaning "to mold or shape". |
| **polyethylene** | The type of plastic commonly used as a liner in the cup of hip replacements. |
| **polymethylmethac-rylate** | The compound that makes up bone cement. |
| **post-traumatic arthritis** | Arthritis that forms in a joint following significant cartilage damage. |
| **prehab** | Physical therapy that occurs before a surgical procedure. |
| **primary care provider** | Also known as a PCP. This is a general practitioner who looks after your overall health condition. This might be a doctor, nurse practitioner, or physician assistant. |
| **prophylaxis** | A treatment given to avoid a known potential complication or disease. |
| **pulmonary embolism** | A blood clot that occurs in the lungs during or after surgery. This complication can be life-threatening. |
| **randomized control trial** | A scientific study wherein the researchers take a treatment, randomly assign that treatment to a group of patients, and gave an alternative or treatment to other patients, and analyze the results. |
| **reamer** | A device used during hip replacement surgery to shape and prepare the acetabulum for the prosthetic cup. |
| **referred pain** | Pain that presents in one part of the body but is generated by a different part of the body. |
| **rheumatoid arthritis** | The most common type of inflammatory arthritis whereby the body attacks its own cells, creating an inflammatory response and wear of cartilage. |

| | |
|---|---|
| **SCD** | An abbreviation for sequential compression device. |
| **sequential compression device** | Pneumatic compression sleeves that squeeze the legs, promoting blood flow and decreasing the risk of blood clots. |
| **severe arthritis** | Severe inflammation or severe cartilage space narrowing in a joint, usually, but not always, associated with severe symptoms. |
| **simultaneous bilateral** | A term that describes having both hips replaced in the same surgical setting, on the same day. |
| **skilled nursing facility** | Also called a SNF (pronounced "sniff"), this is a rehab center where some patients go for full-time care after surgery or an injury. |
| **SNF** | Abbreviation for skilled nursing facility. |
| **staged bilateral** | A term that describes having both hips replaced on different days. The procedures are typically separated by weeks or months. |
| **stem cells** | Cells with the potential to develop into many different types of cells in the body. |
| **stepwise** | Symptoms don't change at a constant rate but get worse, then better, then worse, etc. |
| **steroid** | A class of medications used to decrease inflammation and pain. There are oral and injectable forms. Synonyms include corticosteroid and cortisone. |
| **steroid flare** | An increase in pain that rarely occurs after a steroid injection. This usually resolves with time. |
| **stiffness** | Loss of range of motion in a hip joint caused by underlying arthritis. |
| **supplements** | Non-pharmaceutical dietary aids that are not regulated by the FDA. |

| | |
|---|---|
| **surgical approach** | How a joint is accessed for joint replacement surgery. Different approaches use different incision locations and dive down between different muscular planes. |
| **surgical dressing** | The bandage over the surgical incision. |
| **survivorship** | The lifespan of a hip replacement before failure or revision. |
| **sutures** | A synonym for stitches. |
| **symptomatic relief** | Addressing the symptoms of a disease without fixing the underlying problem or changing the underlying structure. |
| **synergistically** | Two drugs working in a cooperative manner to produce a result greater than either drug would produce individually. |
| **synovial fluid** | Fluid naturally found inside of a joint. |
| **tendons** | Fibrous soft tissue structures that connect muscles to bones. |
| **venous thromboembolism** | A blood clot that occurs in the veins. |
| **viscosupplementation injections** | Hyaluronic acid injections. |
| **VTE** | Abbreviation for venous thromboembolism. |
| **ward** | An area of the hospital where patients stay overnight. |

# Image Credits

| | |
|---|---|
| Figure 2-1 | © [blueringmedia] / Adobe Stock |
| Figure 2-2 | © [blueringmedia] / Adobe Stock |
| Figure 2-3 | © [cbsva / NICOLAS LARENTO] / Adobe Stock |
| Figure 3-1 | © [Spectral-Design] / Adobe Stock |
| Figure 3-2B | © [9nong] / Adobe Stock |
| Figure 3-3A | © [RFBSIP] / Adobe Stock |
| Figure 3-3B | © [WavebreakmediaMicro] / Adobe Stock |
| Figure 5-1 | © [blueringmedia] / Adobe Stock |
| Figure 5-2 | © [bht2000] / Adobe Stock |
| Figure 5-3 | © [blueringmedia] / Adobe Stock with modifications by OrthoSkool Publishing |
| Figure 5-4 | © [denissimonov] / Adobe Stock |
| Figure 5-5 | © [blueringmedia] / Adobe Stock |
| Figure 5-6 | © [glisic_albina] / Adobe Stock |
| Figure 5-7A | Used with permission from Mizuho OSI |
| Figure 5-7B | © AO Foundation, Switzerland (Source: AO surgery reference, www.aosurgery.org) |
| Figure 8-1 | © [Destina] and [Nikolayev]/ Adobe Stock |

Uncredited images were either purchased from stock image sources that do not require crediting for commercial use or were created and owned by OrthoSkool Publishing. No images may be reused without the written consent of the image owner. All images in this book are subject to applicable copyright law.

# Selected References

1. AAOS. *MANAGEMENT OF OSTEOARTHRITIS OF THE HIP: EVIDENCE-BASED CLINICAL PRACTICE GUIDELINE.* 2017; Available from: http://www.orthoguidelines.org/guideline-detail?id=1381.

2. Hochberg, M.C., et al., *American College of Rheumatology 2012 recommendations for the use of nonpharmacologic and pharmacologic therapies in osteoarthritis of the hand, hip, and knee.* Arthritis Care Res (Hoboken), 2012. **64**(4): p. 465-74.

3. Surgeons, A.A.o.H.a.K. *Biologics for Advanced Hip and Knee Arthritis - Position of the American Association of Hip and Knee Surgeons.* Available from: http://www.aahks.org/position-statements/biologics-for-advanced-hip-and-knee-arthritis/.

4. Surgeons, A.A.o.H.a.K. *Opioid Use for the Treatment of Osteoarthritis of the Hip and Knee - Position of the American Association of Hip and Knee Surgeons.* Available from: http://www.aahks.org/position-statements/opioid-use-for-the-treatment-of-osteoarthritis-of-the-hip-and-knee/.

5. Geller, A.I., et al., *Emergency Department Visits for Adverse Events Related to Dietary Supplements.* N Engl J Med, 2015. **373**(16): p. 1531-40.

6. Brown, G.A., *AAOS clinical practice guideline: treatment of osteoarthritis of the knee: evidence-based guideline, 2nd edition.* J Am Acad Orthop Surg, 2013. **21**(9): p. 577-9.

7. Boehnke, K.F. and D.J. Clauw, *Brief Commentary: Cannabinoid Dosing for Chronic Pain Management.* Ann Intern Med, 2019. **170**(2): p. 118.

8. *Cannabidiol (CBD) — what we know and what we don't.* 2018 October 19, 2019]; Available from: https://www.health.harvard.edu/blog/cannabidiol-cbd-what-we-know-and-what-we-dont-2018082414476.

9.  Learmonth, I.D., C. Young, and C. Rorabeck, *The operation of the century: total hip replacement.* Lancet, 2007. **370**(9597): p. 1508-19.

10. Sollecito, T.P., et al., *The use of prophylactic antibiotics prior to dental procedures in patients with prosthetic joints: Evidence-based clinical practice guideline for dental practitioners--a report of the American Dental Association Council on Scientific Affairs.* J Am Dent Assoc, 2015. **146**(1): p. 11-16 e8.

# Do you need more joint replacement education or know someone who does?

Check out these websites for an engaging, interactive, online education experience:

www.OrthoSkool.com

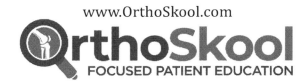

www.KneeSkool.com

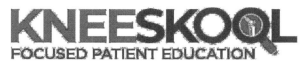

www.HipSkool.com

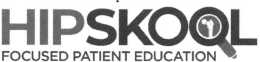

Made in the USA
Middletown, DE
03 November 2019